Essential Questions in Paediatrics for MRCPCH – Volume 2

Edited by

Dr R M Beattie BSc MBBS MRCP FRCPCH
Consultant Paediatric Gastroenterologist
Paediatric Medical Unit
Southampton General Hospital
Southampton

and

Dr M P Champion BSc MBBS MRCP MRCPCH
Consultant in Paediatric Metabolic Medicine
Evelina Children's Hospital
Guy's and St. Thomas' Hospital NHS Trust
London

PASTEST
Dedicated to your success

© 2004 PasTest Ltd
Egerton Court
Parkgate Estate
Knutsford
Cheshire, WA16 8DX

Telephone: 01565 752000

First edition 2004

ISBN: 1 904627 33 1

A catalogue record for this book is available from the British Library.

The information contained within this book was obtained by the authors from reliable sources. However, while every effort has been made to ensure its accuracy, no responsibility for loss, damage or injury occasioned to any person acting or refraining from action as a result of information contained herein can be accepted by the publisher or the authors.

PasTest Revision Books and Intensive Courses

PasTest has been established in the field of postgraduate medical education since 1972, providing revision books and intensive study courses for doctors preparing for their professional examinations. Books and courses are available for the following specialties:

MRCP Part 1 and Part 2, MRCPCH Part 1 and Part 2, MRCOG, DRCOG, MRCGP, MRCPsych, DCH, FRCA, MRCS and PLAB.

For further details contact:

PasTest Ltd, Freepost, Knutsford, Cheshire, WA16 7BR
Tel: 01565 752000   Fax: 01565 650264
Email: enquiries@pastest.co.uk   Web site: www.pastest.co.uk

Typeset by Saxon Graphics Ltd, Derby
Printed by MPG Books Ltd, Bodmin, Cornwall

Contents

Contributors List

Dr R M Beattie BSc MBBS MRCP FRCPCH
Consultant Paediatric Gastroenterologist
Paediatric Medical Unit
Southampton General Hospital
Southampton

Mike Champion BSc MBBS MRCP MRCPCH
Consultant in Paediatric Metabolic Medicine
Evelina Children's Hospital
Guy's and St. Thomas' Hospital NHS Trust
London

Andrew Clark MBBS MRCP MD
Consultant in Paediatric Allergy
Department of Allergy
Addenbrookes NHS Trust
Cambridge

Katy Fidler BSc MBBS MRCPCH
Clinical Research Fellow
Department of Infectious Diseases and Microbiology
Institute of Child Health
London

Grenville F Fox MBChB MRCP FRCPCH
Consultant Neonatologist
Neonatal unit
Guy's and St Thomas' Hospital NHS Trust
London

James W Hart MBBS BSc (Hons) MRCP (UK) MRCPCH
Specialist Registrar
Paediatric Medical Unit
Southampton General Hospital
Southampton

N Hasson MBChB FRCPCH
Consultant in Paediatric Rheumatology
Great Ormond Street Hospital For Children
London

Tammy Hedderly MRCPCH, MBBS, BSc (Hons)
SpR Paediatric Neurology
Department of Paediatric Neurology
Guy's and St Thomas' Hospital NHS Trust
London

Emma J Lim BMBS MSc MRCP
Specialist Registrar in Paediatric Infectious Diseases
Department of Paediatric Infectious Disease
St Mary's Hospital
London

Chris Reid MRCP (UK) FRCPCH
Consultant Paediatric Nephrologist
Department of Paediatric Nephrology and Urology
Guy's and St. Thomas' Hospital NHS Trust
London

Angie M Wade MSc PhD CStat ILTM
Senior Lecturer in Medical Statistics
Centre for Paediatric Epidemiology and Biostatistics
Institute of Child Health
London

Introduction

These revision texts have been written to accompany Essential Revision Notes in Paediatrics for the MRCPCH but are also relevant for part one of the DCH examination. The questions, in the new format are designed to help facilitate revision for the MRCPCH part one examination. The books are split by subject to aid revision planning. Each question has a detailed explanation and so the text can be used as a stand alone revision aid.

The candidate is advised to consult the RCPCH website for up to date information regarding the exam. The information below is taken from the website and is correct at the time of going to press.

The MRCPCH Part One examination consists of two papers.

Paper One A (Basic Child Health) will focus on the areas of child health that are relevant to those who will be working with children in their medical careers, not just those entering mainstream hospital-based paediatrics. The areas to be tested will be those conditions likely to be seen in 6 to 12 months of hospital, community or primary care practice.

Paper One B (Extended Paediatrics) will focus on the more complex paediatric problem-solving skills not tested in Paper One A, and on the scientific knowledge underpinning paediatrics. This is equivalent to the current MRCPCH Part One paper.

Candidates for MRCPCH must successfully complete both Paper One A and One B before being allowed to enter MRCPCH Part Two. .

Paper One A (Basic Child Health) will replace the current Diploma in Child Health (DCH) written papers.

The papers will consist of

Multiple true-false questions used to test knowledge when there is an absolute Yes/No answer.

Best of Five questions used to test judgement and experience. A simple statement or short clinical scenario leads into five options. All could be possible but only one is completely or the most correct. The candidate has to choose the best option.

Extended matching questions (EMQs) are used in the same way as Best of Five questions. In this case a list of 10 possible answers is offered with three statements or clinical scenarios. The candidate chooses the best option from the introductory list. Again, all could be possible but only one is completely or the most correct.

Further details on the make up of the three types of questions are on the college website. There are also downloadable sample papers which should be reviewed.

We are indebted in the production of this book to the many authors who have enthusiastically contributed chapters and to Kirsten Baxter at Pastest for her enthusiasm and expertise in helping pull the book together.

Mark Beattie

Mike Champion

June 2004

Infectious diseases

Katy Fidler and Emma Lim

Multiple Choice Questions

1. The following infections can cause bronchiolitis in infants

- ○ A adenovirus
- ○ B Epstein–Barr virus (EBV)
- ○ C respiratory syncytial virus (RSV)
- ○ D rhinovirus
- ○ E myxovirus

2. Typical features of typhoid fever include

- ○ A persistent pyrexia
- ○ B splenomegaly
- ○ C bradycardia
- ○ D conjunctivitis
- ○ E cough

3. The following are characteristic features of measles

- ○ A diarrhoea
- ○ B fine maculopapular rash starting on the face
- ○ C purulent conjunctivitis
- ○ D convulsions
- ○ E coryza

4. The following organisms are recognised causes of diarrhoea

- ○ A *Enterobacter*
- ○ B rotavirus
- ○ C *Salmonella*
- ○ D enterovirus
- ○ E *Campylobacter*

questions

5. The following skin lesions are caused by viral infections

- A whitlow
- B verruca
- C impetigo
- D tinea capitis
- E molluscum contagiosum

6. The characteristic rash of chickenpox is described as having

- A spots mainly on the hands and feet
- B spots that coalesce
- C spots that are itchy
- D spots appearing in crops
- E spots starting as vesicles

7. Children in the same classroom are at a high risk of catching the following infections from each other

- A human immunodeficiency virus
- B hepatitis C
- C atypical *Mycobacterium*
- D Lyme disease
- E erythema infectiosum

8. The following infections are transmitted by the faeco-oral route

- A rubella
- B polio
- C *Pneumococcus*
- D *Salmonella*
- E Norwalk virus

9. First-line management of infectious diarrhoea in a toddler includes

- A oral rehydration salts
- B metronidazole
- C loperamide
- D kaolin syrup
- E hyoscine butylbromide

10. A 9-month-old child with croup, who has marked stridor at rest and a barking cough, should be treated with

- A nebulised adrenaline (epinephrine)
- B nebulised salbutamol
- C intravenous antibiotics
- D oral dexamethasone or nebulised budesonide
- E intramuscular adrenaline

11. Which of the following complications Is a 12 year old boy with orbital cellulitis at risk of developing?

○ A meningitis
○ B cavernous sinus thrombosis
○ C cerebral abscess
○ D cerebral artery embolus
○ E epistaxis

12. A 1-year-old child presenting with the following conditions would need further investigation of their immune function

○ A herpes stomatitis
○ B cytomegalovirus (CMV) pneumonitis
○ C two previous admissions – one with meningitis, one with pneumonia
○ D six viral upper respiratory infections in 1 year
○ E an atypical mycobacterial skin lesion

13. The following are notifiable diseases

○ A pertussis
○ B malaria
○ C measles
○ D viral meningitis
○ E meningococcal meningitis

14. The following statements about human immunodeficiency virus (HIV) infection in children are correct

○ A most babies are infected by horizontal transmission from their mothers
○ B a baby who is HIV-antibody-positive at 3 months of age is probably infected with HIV
○ C a baby who is HIV-PCR-positive at 3 months of age is probably infected with HIV
○ D most babies who are infected acquire their infection prior to delivery
○ E anti-retroviral therapy should be given to babies of HIV-positive mothers within 12 hours of birth

questions

15. **A 2-year-old presents with a mass in the right side of the neck, thought to be an enlarged cervical lymph node. The following would be included in the differential diagnosis**

- ○ A atypical tuberculosis
- ○ B cat scratch fever
- ○ C lymphoma
- ○ D *Rubella* infection
- ○ E *Toxoplasmosis* infection

16. **The following is true regarding meningitis**

- ○ A hearing impairment is more common after meningococcal than pneumococcal meningitis
- ○ B neck stiffness is a common presenting sign in neonates
- ○ C steroids may reduce the morbidity of *Haemophilus influenzae* type B (Hib) meningitis
- ○ D glucose level in cerebrospinal fluid (CSF) is not usually lowered in tuberculous meningitis
- ○ E *Listeria monocytogenes* is the most common cause of neonatal meningitis

17. **Children with defects in their cellular immune system are particularly at risk of infections with**

- ○ A mycobacteria
- ○ B adenovirus
- ○ C *Staphylococcus aureus*
- ○ D *Pneumocystis carinii*
- ○ E *Neisseria meningitidis*

18. **The following is true of childhood exanthema**

- ○ A the rash of chickenpox characteristically starts behind the ears and along the hairline
- ○ B the rash of measles characteristically starts behind the ears and along the hairline
- ○ C the rash of roseola infantum characteristically gives very erythematous cheeks
- ○ D the rash of roseola infantum characteristically appears after the fever
- ○ E the rash of coxsackie virus characteristically gives vesicular lesions on the hands and feet

19. **The following are proinflammatory cytokines**

- ○ A interleukin-1
- ○ B interleukin-6
- ○ C interleukin-8
- ○ D interleukin-10
- ○ E tumour necrosis factor (TNF)-α

20. The following organisms are Gram stain negative

- ○ A *Bordetella pertussis*
- ○ B *Bacillus anthracis*
- ○ C *Pseudomonas aeruginosa*
- ○ D *Neisseria meningitidis*
- ○ E *Haemophilus influenzae*

21. The following drugs used in the treatment of tuberculosis may cause the side effects described

- ○ A rifampicin and hepatitis
- ○ B ethambutol and deafness
- ○ C isoniazid and peripheral neuropathy
- ○ D streptomycin and deafness
- ○ E pyrazinamide and loss of colour vision

questions

Best Of Five Questions

22. **A 3-year-old girl with vertically acquired HIV has recently started anti-retroviral therapy. Which of the following investigations would be BEST to monitor efficacy of treatment?**

- ○ A CD8 count
- ○ B Full blood count
- ○ C HIV antibody
- ○ D HIV viral load
- ○ E Immunoglobulins

23. **A 6-month-old girl has a proven *Escherichia coli* urine infection. The MOST useful investigation to identify any renal scarring would be?**

- ○ A DMSA (dimercaptosuccinic acid) scan
- ○ B Intravenous pyelogram (IVP)
- ○ C MAG 3 renogram
- ○ D Micturating cystourethrogram (MCUG)
- ○ E Renal ultrasound

24. **A 2-year-old girl presents to casualty with a 24-hour history of being febrile and miserable and has developed a rapidly spreading non-blanching rash. She has cool peripheries and is drowsy. The LEAST useful investigation to do immediately is which of the following?**

- ○ A Blood culture
- ○ B Full blood count
- ○ C Lumbar puncture
- ○ D Meningococcal PCR (polymerase chain reaction)
- ○ E Rapid antigen screen

25. **Which one of the following children does NOT require specific varicella zoster immunoglobulin (VZIG) after being exposed to a case of chickenpox?**

- ○ A A child currently on chemotherapy
- ○ B A child who had a bone marrow transplant 1 month ago
- ○ C A child with a kidney transplant who is on immunosuppressive treatment
- ○ D A child who has had prednisolone 1 mg/kg for the last 6 weeks
- ○ E A child who had prednisolone 2 mg/kg for 3 days 1 week ago

26. An 11-year-old boy presents with a 10-day history of headache, sore throat, chest pain and dry cough. His GP gave him a course of Amoxil 4 days ago but he is no better and is now coughing up yellow sputum and is wheezy. He also complains of abdominal pain and painful swollen knees. Which of the following organisms is MOST likely to be the cause of his illness?

○ A *Streptococcus pneumoniae*
○ B *Mycoplasma pneumoniae*
○ C *Mycobacterium tuberculosis*
○ D *Chlamydia trachomatis*
○ E *Haemophilus influenzae*

27. Which of the following is the MOST likely congenital infection in a baby born with a 'blueberry muffin rash', cataracts, and a heart murmur?

○ A Cytomegalovirus (CMV) infection
○ B Toxoplasmosis infection
○ C Parvovirus infection
○ D HIV infection
○ E Rubella infection

Extended Matching questions

28. Theme: Differential diagnosis of neonatal infection

A *Listeria monocytogenes* infection
B Group A streptococcal infection
C Group B streptococcal (GBS) infection
D Disseminated herpes simplex virus infection
E *Escherichia coli* infection
F Congenital heart disease
G Methylmalonic aciduria
H Congenital infection
I HIV infection

For each of the following case scenarios select the most likely diagnosis from the list above. Each option may be used once, more than once, or not at all.

○ 1. A baby boy presents on day 1 of life with tachypnoea, poor feeding and delayed capillary refill time of 3 seconds. He had been born by normal vaginal delivery (NVD) at 37 weeks, after prolonged rupture of membranes (PROM) for 4 days. Further examination reveals a bulging fontanelle. Initial investigations are as follows (normal ranges in brackets): haemoglobin 14 g/dL (10.5–14 g/dL); white blood cells (WBC) 18 × 10⁹/L (6–15 × 10⁹/L); urea 8 mmol/L (2.5–6.6 mmol/L); creatinine 68 μmol/L (20–80 μmol/L); pH 7.29 (7.32–7.37); bicarbonate (HCO_3^-) 20 mmol/L; carbon dioxide (CO_2) 4.0 kPa; base excess (BE) –6 mmol/L; alanine aminotransferase (ALT) 33 IU/L (10–40 IU/L); prothrombin time (PT) normal; APPT (activated partial PT) normal; C-reactive protein (CRP) 22 (< 5 mg/dL); O_2 saturations in air 97%.

○ 2. A baby girl presents at day 8 of life with tachypnoea, poor feeding and delayed capillary refill time of 4 seconds. She had been born by NVD at 37 weeks after prolonged rupture of membranes for 3 days. Further examination revealed an enlarged liver, easy bruising and a vesicular rash. Initial investigations are as follows: haemoglobin 14 g/dL (10.5–14 g/dL); WBC 8 × 10⁹/L (6–15 × 10⁹/L); urea 8 mmol/L (2.5–6.6 mmol/L); creatinine 68 μmol/L (20–80 μmol/L); pH 7.28 (7.32–7.37); HCO_3^- 19 mmol/L; CO_2 4.0 kPa; BE –9 mmol/L; ALT 787 IU/L (10–40 IU/L); PT grossly abnormal; APPT grossly abnormal; CRP 4 (< 5 mg/dL); O_2 saturations in air 97%.

○ 3. A baby boy presents at day 3 of life with tachypnoea, poor feeding, vomiting and delayed capillary refill time of 4 seconds. He had been born by NVD at 37 weeks with no PROM. Further examination revealed an enlarged liver and lethargy. Initial investigations are as follows: haemoglobin 14 g/dL (10.5–14 g/dL); white blood cells 8 × 10⁹/L (6–15 × 10⁹/L); urea 8 mmol/L (2.5–6.6 mmol/L); creatinine 68 μmol/L (20–80 μmol/L); pH 7.25 (7.32–7.37); HCO_3^- 16 mmol/L; CO_2 3.5 kPa; BE –14 mmol/L; ALT 8 IU/L (10–40 IU/L); PT normal; APPT normal; CRP 4 (< 5 mg/dL); O_2 saturations in air 97%.

29. Theme: Non imported UK infectious diseases

A   Tuberculosis (TB)
B   Hepatitis B
C   Juvenile idiopathic arthritis (JIA)
D   Brucellosis
E   Epstein–Barr virus (EBV)
F   Bacterial osteomyelitis
G   Infective endocarditis
H   Lyme disease
I   Acute lymphoblastic leukaemia (ALL)

For each of the following case scenarios select the most likely diagnosis from the list above. Each option may be used once, more than once, or not at all.

○   1. A 4-year-old boy presents with a 2-week history of fever and being miserable. His mother says he complains of painful joints and muscles and general malaise. She has noticed conjunctivitis and a distinctive rash with large annular erythematous lesions. He has recently been camping in woodland. Initial investigations are as follows (normal ranges in brackets): haemoglobin 11 g/dL (10.5–14 g/dL); WBC 10 × 10^9/L (6–15 × 10^9/L); lymphocytes 4.5 × 10^9/L; neutrophils 6.0 × 10^9/L; eosinophils 0.2 × 10^9/L; urea 3 mmol/L (2.5–6.6 mmol/L); creatinine 45 μmol/L (20–80μmol/L); ALT 30 IU/L (10–40 IU/L); PT normal; APPT normal; CRP 2 (< 5 mg/dL); erythrocyte sedimentation rate (ESR) 30 (< 20 mm/hour).

○   2. A 4-year-old boy presents with a 3-week history of fever and being miserable. His mother says he has been complaining of generalised aches and pains and malaise especially in the right leg and has now developed a limp. He has recently been on holiday in London. X ray of the tibia shows periosteal elevation. Initial investigations are as follows: haemoglobin 10 g/dL (10.5–14 g/dL); WBC 17 × 10^9/L (6–15 × 10^9/L) ; lymphocytes 4.0 × 10^9/L; neutrophils 13.0 × 10^9/L; eosinophils 0.2 × 10^9/L; urea 3 mmol/L (2.5–6.6 mmol/L) ; creatinine 45 μmol/L (20–80μmol/L); ALT 30 IU/L (10–40 IU/L); PT normal; APPT normal; CRP 25 (< 5 mg/dL); ESR 60 (< 20 mm/hour).

○   3. A 4-year-old boy presents with a 3-week history of fever and being miserable. His mother says he is complaining of painful joints and muscles and general malaise. She has noticed an intermittent rash and intermittent arthritis of his knees. Examination also reveals splenomegaly. He has just returned from holiday in Spain. Initial investigations are as follows: haemoglobin 9 g/dL (10.5–14 g/dL); WBC 11 × 10^9/L (6–15 × 10^9/L) ; lymphocytes 4.0 × 10^9/L; neutrophils 6.0 × 10^9/L; eosinophils 0.2 × 10^9/L; platelets 445 × 10^9/L (150–450 × 10^6/L); urea 3 mmol/L (2.5–6.6 mmol/L); creatinine 45 μmol/L (20–80 μmol/L); ALT 30 IU/L (10–40 IU/L); PT normal; APPT normal; CRP 20 (< 5mg/dL); ESR 60 (< 20 mm/hour).

questions (side margin)

30. Theme: Tropical infectious diseases

A   *Giardia*
B   Yellow fever
C   Typhoid
D   Malaria
E   Tuberculosis
F   Diphtheria
G   Tetanus
H   Ebola
I   Dengue fever
J   Human immunodeficiency virus (HIV)

For each of the following case scenarios select the most likely diagnosis from the list above. Each option may be used once, more than once, or not at all.

○ 1. A 4-year-old girl, returned from holiday in India, presents with a 4-week history of swinging fevers, diarrhoea and general malaise, and a rash. Temperature 38°C; pulse 80 beats/min; respiratory rate 15 per min; blood pressure (BP) 100/60 mmHg; ; haemoglobin 10 g/dL (normal range 10.5–14 g/dL); white blood cells (WBC) 6 × 10⁹/L (6–15 × 10⁹/L); platelets 80 × 10⁹/L; neutrophils 2.0 × 10⁹/L; lymphocytes 2.5 × 10⁹/L; eosinophils 0.3 × 10⁹/L (150–400); bilirubin 20 μmol/L (1.7–26μmol/L); aspartate aminotransferase (AST) 80 IU/L (10–45 IU/L); serum sodium 129 mmol/L (135–145 mmol/L); serum potassium 3.7 mmol/L (3.5–5.6 mmol/L); serum urea 6.5 mmol/L (2.5–6.6 mmol/L).

○ 2. A 3-year-old girl, recently arrived from Uganda, presents with a 2-week history of intermittent pyrexia and a 5-week history of persistent diarrhoea, oral thrush and weight loss. Temperature 37.8°C; pulse 70 beats/min; respiratory rate 13 breaths per min; BP 90/56 mmHg; haemoglobin 9.2 g/dL (10.5–14 g/dL); WBC 12 × 10⁹/L (6–15 × 10⁹/L); platelets 100 × 10⁹/L (150–450 × 10⁹/L); neutrophils 9.5 × 10⁹/L; lymphocytes 2.5 × 10⁹/L; eosinophils 0.3 × 10⁹/L; bilirubin 15 μmol/L (1.7–26μmol/L); AST 40 IU/L (10–45 IU/L); serum sodium 136 mmol/L (135–145 mmol/L); serum potassium 3.9 mmol/L (3.5–5.6 mmol/L); serum urea 4.5 mmol/L (2.5–6.6 mmol/L).

○ 3. A 5-year-old who returned from Ghana last week presents with a 2-week history of spiking fevers, vomiting and a cough. Temperature 39° C; pulse 120 beats/min; respiratory rate 20 per min; BP 105/58 mmHg; haemoglobin 7.6 g/dL (10.5–14 g/dL); WBC 10 × 10⁹/L (6–15 × 10⁹/L); platelets 80 × 10⁹/L (150–450 × 10⁹/L); neutrophils 4.0.0 × 10⁹/L; lymphocytes 4.5 × 10⁹/L; eosinophils 0.2 × 10⁹/L; bilirubin 45 μmol/L (1.7–26μmol/L); AST 39 IU/L (10–45 IU/L); serum sodium 131 mmol/L (135–145 mmol/L); serum potassium 4.2 mmol/L (3.5–5.6 mmol/L); serum urea 7.5 mmol/L (2.5–6.6 mmol/L).

answers

1. Bronchiolitis in infants

Answers: A C D E

Bronchiolitis is a common cause of lower respiratory infections in infancy. It causes significant symptoms including cough, wheeze, shortness of breath, and difficulty feeding. About 2% of all infants require hospital admission. The majority of cases (up to 75%) are caused by respiratory syncytial virus (RSV), although adenovirus, rhinovirus and myxovirus can also cause it. Adenovirus can cause a particularly severe illness. Primary Epstein–Barr virus (EBV) infection does not cause a lower respiratory infection but can present as fever, sore throat and cervical lymphadenopathy.

2. Typical features of typhoid fever

Answers: A B C E

Typhoid is known as the great mimic and can present in many ways. Typically children have persistent swinging pyrexia, headache, diarrhoea, vomiting, abdominal pain, and a cough. Characteristic features of typhoid include rose spots (pink macules) and a relative bradycardia when pyrexial. They may also have signs of heart failure, meningism or shock. Splenomegaly is present in around 25% of cases.

3. Features of measles

Answers: B E

Measles characteristically presents with a prodromal illness, which includes coryzal symptoms (runny nose), non-purulent conjunctivitis and cough followed by a rash. Koplik spots appear now (grey white lesions on the buccal mucosa). The typical rash is maculopapular starting on the face and working down the trunk. The lesions tend to coalesce and fade to a dusky colour. Children often have a sore mouth, however diarrhoea is not common. Convulsions are not a characteristic feature of measles and if they occur they are invariably triggered by the fever, or reflect encephalitis.

4. Organisms causing diarrhoea

Answers: B C D E

All can cause diarrhoea except for *Enterobacter*, which is a part of the normal gut flora.

5. Skin lesions caused by viral infections

Answers: A B E

Herpes simplex virus cause whitlow. Human papilloma virus causes verrucae, and molluscum is caused by a virus from the pox family. Impetigo is a bacterial infection, often *Staphylococcus* or *Streptococcus*, and tinea is a fungal infection.

6. Chickenpox rash

Answers: C D

The characteristic rash of chickenpox is a crop of macules which quickly become papular, vesicular, and finally pustular before forming a crust. The rash evolves in a series of crops and lesions of different ages can be seen. The rash is mainly on the trunk but can be seen on the face and limbs. The spots do not coalesce and once they are vesicles they become very itchy.

7. Risk of disease in the classroom

Answer: E

Erythema infectiosum, or slapped cheek or Fifths disease, occurs in outbreaks in primary school children typically during the winter or spring. Human immunodeficiency virus (HIV) is transmitted vertically, sexually or via blood products. Hepatitis C is also vertically and blood acquired. Atypical *Mycobacterium* has a very low infectivity rate between children. Lyme disease is spread by tick bites.

8. Faeco-oral route in disease transmission

Answers: B D E

Polio, *Salmonella* and Norwalk virus are all transmitted by the faeco-oral route and therefore infections are exacerbated by poor hygiene – especially lack of hand washing.

9. Infectious diarrhoea in toddlers

Answer: A

The first-line treatment of diarrhoea in infants is the prevention and treatment of fluid and electrolyte loss by encouraging them to drink. This can be done with an oral rehydration salts, such as Dioralyte. Anti-motility drugs (loperamide), anti-spasmodics (hyoscine) and absorbents (kaolin) are not recommended in children. Simple diarrhoea does not require an antibiotic because it will usually resolve without treatment and is most often caused by viral infection.

10. Croup

Answers: A D

Mild croup (barking cough with no stridor at all) does not require specific treatment. Severe croup (stridor at rest – as opposed to on crying or when distressed) should be treated with oral dexamethasone; if the child refuses or cannot take oral medication this can be given as nebulised budesonide. For severe croup, adrenaline is given in nebulised form rather than intramuscularly. Croup is a viral infection and does not require antibiotics. Moderate croup (stridor on exertion) should be treated with oral or nebulised steroids.

11. Orbital cellulitis

Answers: A B C

There are many serious potential complications from orbital cellulitis. These include involvement of the optic nerve, leading to loss of vision, and intracranial extension of infection, leading to meningitis and intracranial abscesses. Cavernous sinus thrombosis is another well-recognised complication because the venous drainage around the orbit and face is back into the cavernous sinus. Finally, it is always worth imaging the sinuses because orbital cellulitis is often associated with underlying sinusitis.

12. Investigation of immune function

Answers: B C

Herpes stomatitis and atypical mycobacterial skin infections do not require further investigation if they are the only infections a child has had. Cytomegalovirus (CMV) pneumonitis is unusual in children with normal immune function, but children with T cell dysfunction such as HIV can present with this. Any child with two serious bacterial infections needs investigation of their immune system. Finally the occurrence of more than ten to fifteen upper respiratory tract infections in a year may indicate a minor immunodeficiency.

13. Notifiable diseases

Answer: All true

Doctors have a statutory duty to notify a large number of infectious diseases. This helps the implementation of measures to control outbreaks, as well as to continue disease surveillance. Notifiable diseases include:

- Acute encephalitis
- Acute poliomyelitis
- Anthrax
- Cholera
- Diphtheria
- Dysentery
- Food poisoning
- Leptospirosis
- Malaria
- Measles
- Meningitis (meningococcal; pneumococcal; *Haemophilus influenzae*; viral; other specified and unspecified)
- Meningococcal septicaemia
- Mumps
- Ophthalmia neonatorum
- Paratyphoid fever
- Plague
- Rabies
- Relapsing fever
- Rubella
- Scarlet fever
- Smallpox
- Tetanus
- Tuberculosis
- Typhoid fever
- Typhus fever
- Viral haemorrhagic fever
- Viral hepatitis (types A, B, C, and other)
- Whooping cough
- Yellow fever.

14. HIV infection in children

Answers: C E

Most babies are infected by vertical transmission from an HIV-positive mother. Infection usually occurs intrapartum (at delivery), although it may occur prior to delivery or postnatally, especially if breastfeeding. Mother-to-child transmission (MTCT) can be reduced from approximately 30% to less than 1% with the following measures:

- Anti-retroviral therapy (ART) to mother in pregnancy to get viral load < 50 copies/mL
- ART to baby for the first 4–6 weeks of life
- Delivery by lower segment caesarian section (LSCS), ensuring no prolonged rupture of membranes (if possible)
- Avoidance of breastfeeding.

Babies should be diagnosed by polymerase chain reaction (PCR), or viral culture if under 18 months of age, as maternal antibody may persist this long and so give false-positive results. It is important to give anti-retroviral therapy as soon as possible after birth.

15. Enlarged cervical lymph node

Answers: A B C E

A, B, C and E may present with cervical lymphadenopathy. Atypical tuberculosis is usually unilateral and painless, and often long-standing. Cat scratch fever is caused by the organism *Bartonella henselae*, a Gram-negative bacterium that is transmitted by cats (usually kittens) to humans by a scratch or a bite. Of those infected, 30% experience a fever and mild systemic symptoms but the predominant sign is regional lymphadenopathy involving nodes that drain the site of inoculation. Most disease is self-limiting but if the child is very unwell consider antibiotics such as ciprofloxacin. Rubella characteristically causes post-auricular and sub-occipital lymphadenopathy. Malignancy should always be suspected.

16. Meningitis

Answer: C

Hearing impairment occurs in < 5% of cases of meningitis, overall, and is most common after pneumococcal infection. Neck stiffness occurs in older children only. Neonates present with non-specific signs of infection but may have fullness of their fontanelle. Studies have shown a reduction of deafness and neurological morbidity after Hib meningitis if steroids were given early in the disease course (before or with antibiotics). CSF glucose is usually very low in tuberculous meningitis. Although *Listeria* is a cause of neonatal meningitis, the commonest cause is group B *Streptococcus*.

answers

17. Infection risk in cellular immune system defects

Answers: A B D

Children with defects in their cellular immune system are particularly at risk from intracellular bacteria, such as mycobacteria and *Listeria*, viruses, fungi and opportunistic pathogens such as *Pneumocystis*. Those with antibody defects are more at risk of Gram-positive bacteria, such as *Staphylococcus aureus* and the streptococcal species, as well as some viruses (eg enterovirus). Neutrophil defects are associated with Gram-positive bacterial and fungal infections. Recurrent neisserial infections are classically seen with complement deficiencies.

18. Childhood exanthemas

Answers: B D E

The rash of chickenpox characteristically starts on the trunk. The rash of measles does characteristically start behind the ears and along the hairline as a macular rash. It then becomes maculopapular and spreads sequentially down the body – to the face, the upper arms, trunk and then the legs. It is the rash of parvovirus B19 (erythema infectiosum) that causes the 'slapped cheek' appearance. The rash of roseola infantum is caused by human herpes virus (HHV)-6 and usually appears abruptly when the fever stops. Coxsackie virus, especially type A16, causes 'hand, foot and mouth' disease with intra-oral ulcerative lesions, and vesicular lesions on the hands and feet.

19. Proinflammatory cytokines

Answers: A B E

Cytokines are soluble small proteins that mediate signalling between cells. They usually act in an autocrine (on the cell that produced them) or paracrine (on cells close by) manner. They act by binding to specific receptors at the cell membrane which causes intracellular signalling and the subsequent induction, enhancement, or inhibition of cytokine-regulated genes in the nucleus. Cytokines released at the earliest stages of an infection help to determine the nature of the subsequent immune response and may be described as 'pro' or 'anti' inflammatory.

20. Gram stain negative organisms

Answers: C D E

The Gram stain is a standard method for visualising bacteria by microscopy. The purple stain is retained in the cell wall of Gram-positive organisms, such as staphylococci and streptococci, but is washed out during the staining procedure to a pink colour in Gram-negative bacteria such *Escherichia coli* and other coliforms.

21. Side effects of tuberculosis drugs

Answers: A C D

Standard therapy for tuberculosis now usually consists of four drugs: rifampicin, isoniazid, pyrazinamide and ethambutol (in older children). Rifampicin is associated with hepatitis; isoniazid with a peripheral neuropathy preventable by concurrent pyridoxine therapy; pyrazinamide causes gastritis; and ethambutol causes impairment of visual acuity and colour vision. Eye tests are routinely recommended on starting ethambutol therapy, although this is difficult in younger children.

22. D: HIV viral load

Anti-retroviral treatment is monitored by looking at the CD4 count and the HIV viral load. HIV antibodies may be used in diagnosing HIV infection, however children under 18 months may still have maternally acquired HIV antibodies. High immunoglobulin levels are a non-specific sign that occur in HIV infection. Viral load is *not* the same as HIV antigen as the latter only detects if antigen is present or not; viral load looks at the quantitative amount of HIV virus in the blood and is measured in copies/mL. Less than 50 copies/mL is also known as 'undetectable' and is a sign that the HIV virus is being successfully suppressed by medication (not eradicated, as anti-retroviral therapy is only able to suppress viral replication).

23. A: DMSA scan

DMSA scan is the best test for looking at renal scarring. Intravenous pyelograms (IVPs) are used to look for stones. Renal ultrasound is used to look at the kidney structure, for example, to identify horseshoe or duplex kidneys. Micturating cystourethrogram (MCUG) looks for vesicoureteric reflux. A MAG 3 renogram looks at renal perfusion, not scarring.

24. C: Lumbar puncture

In a shocked child with a history and clinical picture of meningococcaemia the correct management would be to get intravenous access, collect blood for culture, PCR, serology and rapid antigen screen, FBC, clotting, urea and electrolytes (U&Es), and glucose – if insufficient blood is available then the blood cultures and BM stick (glucose) and blood gases and electrolytes are most important initially. Immediate treatment is with oxygen, fluid resuscitation and high-dose intravenous antibiotics. In this scenario, doing a lumbar puncture is very dangerous and could precipitate circulatory collapse. For confirmed meningococcal disease a lumbar puncture is not necessary as it does not alter treatment (7 days of appropriate antibiotics, usually ceftriaxone) for sepsis and/or meningitis. For other causes of meningitis (eg pneumococcal), an abnormal lumbar puncture would lengthen treatment and therefore should be done when the patient is clinically stable. Remember, cell changes persist even after antibiotics have been given.

answers

25. E: A child who had prednisolone 2 mg/kg for 3 days 1 week ago

The following children need VZIG:

- Those on chemotherapy or radiotherapy, or within 6 months of treatment with these
- Those within 6 months of having had a bone marrow transplant
- Those who have had an organ transplant and are on immunosuppressive treatment
- Those who have received within the last 3 months oral prednisolone at more than 1 mg/kg/day for 1 month or 2 mg/kg/day for more than 1 week
- Those who are on steroids in combination with cytotoxic drugs.

Note that this means that a child receiving the standard 3-day course of steroids for an acute exacerbation of asthma would not require VZIG after exposure to chickenpox.

26. B: *Mycoplasma pneumoniae*

This is a typical description of *Mycoplasma pneumoniae*. The history is too short for tuberculosis. *Streptococcus* and *Haemophilus* do not give the extra-pulmonary symptoms and *Chlamydia* causes a chest infection in babies aged 4–6 weeks.

27. E: Rubella infection

Rubella is the most likely diagnosis with this constellation of signs. Toxoplasmosis occasionally may produce cataracts, but is not likely to result in heart defects and murmurs. Symptomatic parvovirus infection usually results in hydrops, anaemia and cardiac failure with a murmur, but no cataracts or blueberry muffin (petechial) rash.

28. DIFFERENTIAL DIAGNOSIS OF NEONATAL INFECTION

1.   C – Group B streptococcal (GBS) infection

This scenario describes the classical early presentation of GBS septicaemia with meningitis. This disease usually present early (< 72 hours) or late (> 8–28 days). There is often a history of PROM, as with many neonatal infections. Blood gas analysis reveals a mild, partially compensated, metabolic acidosis consistent with sepsis. Liver function tests (LFTs) and clotting are normal. CRP is raised in this case although this may not occur in neonates with infection. Other diagnoses in order of likelihood are as follows: *Escherichia coli* infection (may present with early or late disease); *Listeria monocytogenes* infection (may present with early or late disease); Group A streptococcal infection (very rare these days).

2.   D – Disseminated herpes simplex virus infection

Again, as usual in clinical practice, the neonate presents with non-specific signs and symptoms of sepsis. In this case the baby is a little older, has an enlarged liver and grossly abnormal LFTs and clotting. White blood count and

CRP are normal suggesting a non-bacterial cause, however the prolonged rupture of membranes (PROM) gives a clue to an infective cause. The rash is actually vesicular and the baby has disseminated herpes simplex virus (HSV) infection. This classically presents around this time, usually in a mother who has acquired HSV late in the third trimester (often an asymptomatic infection in the mother). Approximately 85% of neonatal HSV infections are acquired at delivery, 5% pre-natally and 10% post-natally (eg from cold sores, herpetic whitlow). Without early treatment with intravenous aciclovir the mortality is extremely high. Other diagnoses, in order of likelihood, are as follows: metabolic disease; overwhelming bacterial sepsis (still the most *common* neonatal diagnosis even if not the most likely in this case); congenital infection. Congenital heart disease may give poor feeding and enlarged liver but not grossly abnormal LFTs or deranged clotting.

3. G – Methylmalonic aciduria

There is no history of PROM, a normal WBC and CRP suggesting non-infective cause. The blood gas reveals severe metabolic acidosis, with mildly raised LFTs making metabolic disease the most likely. This child needs a metabolic work-up although initial management should also cover initially for sepsis with antibiotics. Other diagnoses in order of likelihood in this scenario are as follows: HSV infection; overwhelming bacterial sepsis (still the most *common* neonatal diagnosis even if not the most likely in this case).

29. NON-IMPORTED UK INFECTIOUS DISEASES

1. H – Lyme disease

This is the classical description of Lyme disease, with erythema chronicum migrans rash, especially with a travel history of an area known to have ticks. Lyme disease is caused by the organism *Borrelia burgdorferi* which is transmitted to man by the *Ixodes* tick. If not treated at this primary stage Lyme disease will progress to stages 2 and 3 with further complications. The clinical manifestations of the three stages are:

- Stage 1 (early localised): distinctive rash; erythema migrans; red macule/papule at site of tick bite, which expands over days or weeks to a large annular erythematous lesion with partial clearing, approximately 15 cm diameter; associated with fever, malaise, headache, neck stiffness
- Stage 2 (early disseminated): 3–5 weeks post-bite; multiple erythema migrans; cranial nerve palsies especially VIIth (Bell's); meningitis; conjunctivitis; arthralgia; myalgia; headache; malaise; rarely carditis
- Stage 3 (late disease): recurrent arthritis; pauciarticular, large joints; neuropathy; encephalopathy.

The second option is juvenile idiopathic arthritis (JIA). Systemic onset JIA presents with prolonged fever and malaise but a very different salmon pink rash. The rash of infective endocarditis (IE) (third choice) is also very different with Janeway lesions, splinter haemorrhages and Osler's nodes.

answers

2.   F – Bacterial osteomyelitis

High CRP, white blood cells and ESR with characteristic X-ray changes make this diagnosis the most likely answer – the most common culprit, in an immunologically normal host, is *Staphylococcus aureus*. Osteomyelitis is two to four times more common in boys. Tuberculosis (TB) is the second choice, which can cause osteomyelitis. It is always important to think of malignancy in patients with bony pain, either localized osteosarcoma or acute lymphocytic leukaemia (ALL). Evidence of these would usually be seen with cytopenias on the FBC (full blood count). The third possibility is JIA.

3.   C – Juvenile idiopathic arthritis (JIA)

It is always important to remember non-infectious diseases that present to the infectious diseases department with prolonged fever. This is a classical case of systemic onset juvenile arthritis, with a 'salmon pink' intermittent rash. Splenomegaly can also occur in other diseases such as ALL (but no cytopenia), brucellosis (does not give this rash; no night sweats) and infective endocarditis (no murmur in this case). Cases of *Brucella* can be found in Spain, but of course a travel history is often just incidental. The second possibility is brucellosis, and the third is infective endocarditis.

30. TROPICAL INFECTIOUS DISEASES

1.   C – Typhoid

Typhoid typically presents with a relative bradycardia to the pyrexia. Often the eosinophils and platelets are low. AST can be raised and hyponatraemia is common. With this long history, HIV has to be considered (second choice). Malaria must be excluded but does not usually cause diarrhoea.

2.   J – Human immunodeficiency virus (HIV)

HIV is most likely. Second choice is *Giardia* infection; and third, typhoid. HIV has a longer course and persistent diarrhoea can be a presenting feature. These children can be lymphopenic and thrombocytopenic. Chronic giardiasis can present with offensive stools and a low-grade pyrexia and weight loss; however the blood results do not fit. Typhoid is in the differential, but the patient is not bradycardic and has a normal sodium.

3.   D – Malaria

A child with malaria can present acutely unwell, often with a fever and cough. Severe diarrhoea is rare. They are often anaemic with a raised bilirubin but normal liver function tests. Tuberculosis is the second possibility – although less likely as the history is relatively short. Typhoid is a great mimic of other diseases, and is the third choice.

Metabolic medicine

Mike Champion

Multiple Choice Questions

1. The following inborn errors of metabolism have X-linked recessive inheritance

- ◯ A Hurler syndrome
- ◯ B ornithine transcarbamylase deficiency
- ◯ C biotinidase deficiency
- ◯ D Lesch–Nyhan syndrome
- ◯ E acute intermittent porphyria

2. Hyperlactataemia is a recognised feature of

- ◯ A isovaleric acidaemia
- ◯ B very long chain acyl-co-A dehydrogenase deficiency (VLCAD)
- ◯ C venepuncture with tourniquet
- ◯ D Smith–Lemli–Opitz syndrome
- ◯ E hypovolaemic shock

3. Causes of metabolic acidosis include

- ◯ A hyperammonaemia
- ◯ B chloridorrhoea
- ◯ C maple syrup urine disease
- ◯ D non-ketotic hyperglycinaemia
- ◯ E cystinosis

4. Hypoglycaemia

- ◯ A can be diagnosed by Glucostix
- ◯ B is defined as a glucose concentration of less than 2.0 mmol/L
- ◯ C with the presence of ketones in the urine excludes medium chain acyl-CoA dehydrogenase (MCAD) deficiency as the cause
- ◯ D in the absence of ketones and a glucose requirement greater than 8 mg/kg/min to maintain normoglycaemia, is indicative of hyperinsulinism
- ◯ E secondary to glibenclamide poisoning is associated with a high ratio of insulin to C-peptide

5. The following treatments and conditions are correctly paired

- A methylmalonic acidaemia and glycine
- B tyrosinaemia and betaine
- C Gaucher's disease and bone marrow transplantation
- D ornithine transcarbamylase deficiency and sodium phenylbutyrate
- E non-ketotic hyperglycinaemia and dextromethorphan

6. The following features are common to both Marfan syndrome and classical homocystinuria

- A osteoporosis
- B span is greater than height
- C thrombotic tendency
- D hypermobile joints
- E ectopia lentis

7. Recognised features of cystinuria include

- A photophobia
- B growth faltering
- C renal calculi
- D seizures
- E rickets

8. Phenylketonuria (PKU)

- A breastfeeding is contraindicated in the newborn infant with phenylketonuria
- B the diet is phenylanine-free
- C the concentration of brain phenylalanine directly correlates with that in the plasma
- D 'diet' drinks (with artificial sweeteners) improve phenylalanine control
- E phenylalanine is teratogenic

9. Causes of hyperammonaemia include

- A urinary tract infection
- B argininosuccinic aciduria
- C methylmalonic acidaemia
- D patent ductus venosus
- E liver failure

10. The following are true of mitochondrial DNA

- A replication is inhibited by zidovudine
- B rearrangements have a low risk of recurrence in siblings
- C encodes subunits for all the respiratory chain complexes
- D has no histone coat
- E is inherited from the mother

11. Conjugated hyperbilirubinaemia is a feature of

- ○ A Gilbert syndrome
- ○ B galactosaemia
- ○ C Crigler-Najjar syndrome
- ○ D mitochondrial DNA depletion syndrome
- ○ E tyrosinaemia

12. Metabolic disorders presenting with dysmorphic features in the neonatal period include

- ○ A congenital disorders of glycosylation (CDG) Ia
- ○ B medium chain acyl-coA dehydrogenase (MCAD) deficiency
- ○ C Hurler syndrome
- ○ D Zellweger syndrome
- ○ E Smith–Lemli–Opitz syndrome

13. The following are true concerning cholesterol

- ○ A those at risk of familial hypercholesterolaemia should be screened at birth
- ○ B cholesterol-lowering margarines are effective in the paediatric age group
- ○ C statins are contraindicated in children
- ○ D a low level of high-density lipoprotein (HDL) cholesterol is a risk factor for premature ischaemic heart disease
- ○ E girls are at lower risk than boys for developing premature ischaemic heart disease

14. The following metabolic processes occur within the peroxisome

- ○ A urea cycle
- ○ B fatty acid oxidation
- ○ C glycosylation of glycoproteins
- ○ D bile acid synthesis
- ○ E phytanate oxidation

15. The following are consistent with a diagnosis of propionic acidaemia

- ○ A hyperglycaemia
- ○ B neutropenia
- ○ C hypercalcaemia
- ○ D ketonuria
- ○ E raised lactate

questions

Best of Five Questions

16. **A 10-month-old girl presents with pneumonia. She was noted to have marked hepatomegaly. Before starting intravenous fluids the laboratory glucose was 2.1 mmol/L. Further investigations revealed lactate of 6.1 mmol/L (normal < 2.0), triglycerides of 17 mmol/L (normal < 2.3), and urate of 3.6 mmol/L (normal < 0.47). The MOST likely diagnosis is which of the following?**

   - ○ A Phosphofructokinase deficiency (GSD V)
   - ○ B Glucose-6-phosphatase deficiency (GSD I)
   - ○ C Branching enzyme deficiency (GSD IV)
   - ○ D Debrancher enzyme deficiency (GSD III)
   - ○ E Myophosphorylase deficiency (GSD VII)

17. **An 11-month-old girl was admitted following an afebrile seizure. Urine was negative for ketones on dipstick. Blood glucose was noted to be 1.8 mmol/L. A repeat glucose was 2.6 mmol/L 30 minutes later following a 10% dextrose bolus, and an infusion of 12.5% dextrose was required to maintain normoglycaemia. Further investigations included lactate 1.8 μmol/L (normal < 2), and ammonia 92 μmol/L (normal < 50). What is the NEXT treatment of choice?**

   - ○ A Hydrocortisone
   - ○ B Octreotide
   - ○ C Glucagon
   - ○ D Sub-total pancreatectomy
   - ○ E Diazoxide

18. **A 48-hour-old infant on the post-natal ward is noted to be tachypnoeic, sleepy and feeding poorly. Blood gas analysis shows: pH 7.48; PaO_2 12.3; $PaCO_2$ 3.6; standard bicarbonate 20.0; base excess 1.6. What is the NEXT key investigation?**

   - ○ A Ammonia
   - ○ B Lactate
   - ○ C Chest X-ray
   - ○ D Amino acids
   - ○ E Blood culture

19. An 8-month-old infant was noted to have a metabolic acidosis when being investigated for failure to thrive despite dietary supplementation and no evidence of malabsorption. Ammonia 36 µmol/L (normal < 50), lactate 1.3 µmol/L (normal < 2), anion gap 19. Urinary ketones negative. The MOST likely diagnosis is which of the following?

   ○ A Propionic acidaemia
   ○ B Citrullinaemia
   ○ C Renal tubular acidosis
   ○ D Protein-losing enteropathy
   ○ E Medium chain acyl-CoA dehydrogenase (MCAD) deficiency

20. An infant with microcephaly born to a 36-year-old woman is currently under investigation for potential causes. To exclude maternal phenylketonuria (PKU) what is the investigation of choice?

   ○ A Infant plasma amino acids
   ○ B Maternal plasma amino acids
   ○ C Infant urinary amino acids
   ○ D Maternal urinary organic acids
   ○ E Maternal urinary amino acids

21. An 11-month-old boy presented with an early morning seizure. He had been unwell with gastroenteritis and poor oral intake for 36 hours. His glucose concentration on admission was 1.1 mmol/L. Urinalysis was negative for glucose and ketones. Subsequent organic acid analysis revealed a dicarboxylic aciduria. Which of the following would be the MOST useful investigation?

   ○ A Fat oxidation studies on fibroblasts
   ○ B Acylcarnitines
   ○ C Genotyping for medium chain acyl-CoA dehydrogenase (MCAD) deficiency
   ○ D Amino acids
   ○ E Very long chain fatty acids

22. A 12-month-old girl was referred for investigation for developmental regression having lost the ability to sit unsupported. Examination revealed a cherry red spot. There were no audible murmurs and the abdomen was soft with no palpable organomegaly. What is the MOST likely diagnosis?

   ○ A Fabry disease
   ○ B Sandhoff disease
   ○ C Niemann–Pick type C
   ○ D Gaucher's disease
   ○ E Tay–Sachs disease

Extended Matching Questions

23. Theme: Investigations of inborn errors

A   Very long chain fatty acids
B   Urinary sulphite dipstick
C   Urinary amino acids
D   Plasma amino acids
E   Organic acids
F   Acylcarnitines
G   Urate
H   Lactate
I   Ammonia
J   7–Dehydrocholesterol

For each of the following inborn errors, select the most appropriate initial investigation from the list above. Each option may be used once, more than once, or not at all.

○   1. Zellweger syndrome.
○   2. Maple syrup urine disease (MSUD).
○   3. Lesch–Nyhan syndrome.

24. Theme: Eye signs in inborn errors

A   Ectopia lentis
B   Corneal clouding
C   Stellate iris
E   Pigmentary retinopathy
F   Cherry red spot
G   Cataract
H   Arcus juvenilis
I   Kayser–Fleischer ring
J   Glaucoma

For each of the following inborn errors, select from the list above the eye signs commonly associated with each condition. Each option may be used once, more than once, or not at all.

○   1. Long chain hydroxy acyl-CoA dehydrogenase deficiency.
○   2. Galactosaemia.
○   3. Morquio syndrome.

25. Theme: Liver failure

A   Isovaleric acidaemia
B   Fructosuria
C   Tyrosinaemia
D   Wilson disease
E   Galactosaemia
F   Zellweger syndrome
G   Medium chain acyl-CoA dehydrogenase (MCAD) deficiency
H   Ornithine transcarbamylase (OTC) deficiency
I   Hereditary fructose intolerance

For each of the following case scenarios select the most likely diagnosis from the list above. Each option may be used once, more than once, or not at all.

○ 1. A 5-day-old breast-fed infant with deepening jaundice, gross hepatomegaly and severe bruising. Red reflexes are present. Glucose 3.1 mmol/L. Ammonia 97 μmol/L (normal < 50). INR 5.1. Septic screen: positive blood culture for *Escherichia coli.* Organic acids: elevated phenyllactate and 4–hydroxyphenyllactate. Orotic acid 3.4 mmol/mol creatinine (normal < 5).

○ 2. A 2-day-old formula-fed infant with jaundice, gross hepatomegaly and bruising. Red reflexes are present. Glucose 3.0 mmol/L. Ammonia 117 μmol/L (normal < 50). INR 4.1. Septic screen: negative. Organic acids: increased phenyllactate, 4–hydroxyphenyllactate and succinylacetone. Orotic acid 4.6 mmol/mol creatinine (normal < 5).

○ 3. A 5-month-old infant fed on soya-based formula and first-weaning foods, with recent onset of poor feeding and recurrent vomiting, firm hepatomegaly and marked tachypnoea. Red reflexes are present. Glucose 3.3 mmol/L. Ammonia 82 μmol/L (normal < 50). INR 4.6. Septic screen: negative. Organic acids: increased phenyllactate and 4–hydroxyphenyllactate. Orotic acid 4.9 mmol/mol creatinine (normal < 5).

answers

1. Inborn errors of metabolism

Answers: B D

Inborn errors of metabolism are most commonly inherited in an autosomal recessive fashion. X-linked recessive exceptions include ornithine transcarbamylase (OTC) deficiency, Lesch–Nyhan syndrome, Fabry disease, Hunter syndrome, and adrenoleukodystrophy. Female carriers may have symptoms with OTC due to the effects of lyonisation. Acute intermittent porphyria is inherited in a dominant fashion.

2. Hyperlactataemia

Answers: A B C E

Elevated lactate is a feature of a number of inborn errors including organic acidaemias (A), fat oxidation defects (B), respiratory chain disorders, pyruvate disorders, disorders of gluconeogenesis, hereditary fructose intolerance, biotinidase deficiency, and glycogen storage disorders (I, III, VI and IX). In practice, hypoperfusion and hypoxia need to be excluded because secondary causes of lactic acidaemia are more common. Spurious elevations of lactate commonly arise due to a squeezed blood sample. An arterial sample should be taken if a free-flowing venous sample cannot be obtained. Smith–Lemli–Opitz syndrome is a disorder of cholesterol synthesis resulting in dysmorphism and mental retardation.

3. Metabolic acidosis

Answers: C E

Maple syrup urine disease (MSUD) produces a metabolic acidosis due to the build-up of a number of organic acids. Cystinosis results in damage to the proximal tubule due to cystine storage resulting in a renal tubular acidosis. Non-ketotic hyperglycinaemia (NKH) produces a respiratory acidosis as apnoeas develop. Ammonia is a respiratory stimulant and therefore produces a respiratory alkalosis. Chloridorrhoea produces a metabolic alkalosis secondary to chloride loss in the stool.

4. Hypoglycaemia

Answer: D

Stick tests are used as screens for hypoglycaemia, but may be unreliable at low glucose concentrations. Diagnosis requires formal laboratory confirmation. Hypoglycaemia is defined as a laboratory glucose of ≤ 2.6 mmol/L. Fat oxidation detects such as MCAD are causes of hypoketotic hypoglycaemia, however the ketone production is inappropriately low for the degree of hypoglycaemia, rather than absent. Hyperinsulinism is a further cause of hypoketotic hypoglycaemia characterised by a persistently elevated glucose requirement (> 8 mg/kg/min). Poisoning with exogenous insulin is characterised by a high insulin to C-peptide ratio as the C-peptide is inappropriately low. However, anti-diabetics such as glibenclamide promote endogenous insulin release and so the ratio is normal.

5. Pairing of treatments and conditions

Answers: D E

Organic acids conjugate with glycine and carnitine, speeding their excretion via the kidney. Glycine is used to treat isovaleric acidaemia, whereas carnitine is used in methylmalonic and propionic acidaemias. Tyrosinaemia is treated with NTBC which effectively blocks the production of damaging metabolites in the tyrosine catabolic pathway. The pathway remains blocked, and therefore a low-tyrosine diet is still required, but the hepatic and renal complications are abolished. Betaine is used to re-methylate homocysteine to methionine in classical homocystinuria and in other metabolic blocks with associated elevated homocysteine, eg cobalamin (vitamin B_{12}) defects. Gaucher's disease is a sphingolipidosis characterised by the storage of cerebroside in liver, spleen and nervous system, secondary to glucocerebrosidase deficiency. Previously bone-marrow transplantation has been used, but has been superseded by enzyme replacement therapy. Sodium phenylbutyrate and sodium benzoate are used in urea cycle defects, such as ornithine transcarbamylase deficiency, as an alternate pathway for nitrogen clearance. Conjugation with glutamine and glycine produces water-soluble products that can be excreted directly by the kidney, avoiding the need for processing by the urea cycle, and thus reducing the load on the pathway. Dextromethorphan is a partial antagonist of the NMDA receptor to which glycine binds in the central nervous system. This blocks the excitatory effect of glycine and therefore helps reduce seizures in non-ketotic hyperglycinaemia (NKH). Long-term neurological development remains severely affected.

6. Marfan syndrome and homocystinuria

Answers: B E

Both conditions appear physically similar with a marfanoid habitus, and dislocated lenses. There are differences in the joints, which are stiff in homocystinuria but hypermobile in Marfan syndrome. Intelligence is reduced in homocystinuria. Cardiovascular compromise in Marfan syndrome includes aortic root dilatation, whereas homocystinuria is complicated by thromboses. Osteoporosis is common in homocystinuria, but not in Marfan syndrome.

7. Cystinuria

Answer: C

Cystinuria is a transport defect resulting in the excessive loss of COAL (cystine, ornithine, arginine and lysine) in the urine. The only clinical consequence is renal stone formation. All the listed features are seen in cystinosis. This is a lysosomal defect with excess cystine being stored, with adverse effects on kidneys, liver, thyroid, pancreas and brain.

8. Phenylketonuria

Answer: E

PKU results from a block in phenylalanine metabolism resulting in elevated phenylalanine levels and neurological impairment. It is managed with a phenylalanine-restricted diet. Phenylalanine is an essential amino acid and therefore cannot be totally removed from the diet. In the neonate this can be given as formula or breast milk. The level of phenylalanine in the brain cannot be predicted from the plasma concentration which explains why some patients have good outcomes despite poor control and vice versa. A reduction in transport across the blood brain barrier is protective. 'Diet' drinks are contraindicated because aspartame contains phenylalanine, thus the full sugar varieties are preferred. Phenylalanine is teratogenic, and therefore even though the chance of a PKU mother having a PKU affected child is only 1 in 100, the fetus can still be damaged by maternal PKU. The condition must be managed very carefully in pregnancy, by more frequent blood monitoring and stricter control of phenylalanine concentrations.

9. Hyperammonaemia

Answer: All true

Hyperammonaemia is the hallmark of primary urea cycle defects such as argininosuccinic aciduria. The liver is the home of the urea cycle, and therefore liver failure can result in severe hyperammonaemia. Secondary inhibition of the urea cycle occurs in the organic acidaemias. Transient hyperammonaemia of the newborn is thought to occur when there is delayed closure of the ductus venosus, whereby blood is shunted away from the liver, thus bypassing the urea cycle. Urinary tract infections with urea-splitting organisms (such as proteus) result in the release of ammonia from urea, and are a cause of hyperammonaemia.

10. Mitochondrial DNA

Answer: A B D E

Mitochondrial DNA (mtDNA) is inherited from the maternal egg. The paternal mtDNA is located in the tail of the sperm (which does not enter the egg at fertilisation). Point mutations are inherited through the female line, however rearrangements such as deletions and duplications tend to be sporadic with low risk of recurrence. The mutation rate in mtDNA is higher than nuclear DNA (nDNA), because there is neither a protective histone coat nor the same repair mechanisms enjoyed by DNA within the nucleus. Mitochondria are the product of two genomes, mitochondrial and nuclear. mtDNA does not encode for all the subunits of the respiratory chain complexes. Complex II is entirely nDNA encoded. mtDNA replication is inhibited by nucleoside analogues such as zidovudine. There is some concern about its use in treating pregnant mothers to block the vertical transmission of human immunodeficiency virus (HIV).

11. Conjugated hyperbilirubinaemia

Answers: B D E

Conjugated hyperbilirubinaemia occurs in most inborn errors that adversely affect the liver including galactosaemia and tyrosinaemia. mtDNA depletion syndrome is a nDNA encoded respiratory chain disorder that is associated with severe liver disease in some cases. The mtDNA is qualitatively normal, but reduced in amount. Causes of unconjugated hyperbilirubinaemia include haemolytic anaemia, Crigler–Najjar syndrome and Gilbert syndrome.

12. Dysmorphic features

Answers: A D E

Dysmorphic features occur in inborn errors associated with the making and breaking of complex molecules. Inability to synthesise structural molecules interferes with embryogenesis (eg plasmalogens in Zellweger syndrome, glycoproteins in carbohydrate-deficient glycoprotein syndromes (CDG), and cholesterol in Smith–Lemli–Opitz syndrome). Inability to break down complex molecules (as in lysosomal storage disorders like Hurler syndrome) results in coarse dysmorphic features which develop over time because of accumulated storage. Initially the neonate appears normal. Most patients with inborn errors are not dysmorphic.

13. Cholesterol metabolism

Answers: B D E

At-risk family members should be screened, but ideally not before 5 years of age. This practice is based on the unreliability of neonatal values in predicting adult values, and the lack of evidence to support infant treatment. 'Lifestyle' is the treatment of choice for heterozygotes aged less than 10 years, involving a healthy diet and exercise. The cholesterol-lowering margarines are effective in children and are more palatable than binding resins. Statins are used in children who are homozygotes, and in heterozygotes aged more than 10 years. The age at which to start statins is controversial, and is based on an assessment of cholesterol level, gender, and family history. Girls are at less risk, tending to develop heart disease 10 years later than males. Family

answers

history is a very important independent risk factor for premature heart disease, and is more significant than the degree of hypercholesterolaemia. Low HDL cholesterol is a risk factor for premature ischaemic heart disease.

14. Peroxisome metabolism

Answers: B D E

Peroxisomes are present in all cells except mature red cells. They have many synthetic and catabolic functions. They are the site of biosynthesis of plasmalogens, bile acids, and cholesterol. They are the site of β-oxidation of very long chain and branched chain fatty acids. Other oxidative processes include those of phytanate (vitamin A), glutaric acid, and pipecolic acid. They are also the site for glyoxylate metabolism. Peroxisomal disorders may result from a complete absence of function (Zellweger syndrome), from loss of a few processes, or from blockage of a single pathway, such as phytanate in Refsum disease, and VLCFA oxidation in adrenoleukodystrophy. The urea cycle occurs in the cytoplasm and mitochondrion, and glycosylation of glycoproteins occurs in the endoplasmic reticulum and Golgi. Disorders of this pathway lead to the congenital disorders of glycosylation (CDG).

15. Propionic acidaemia

Answers: A B D E

Propionic acidaemia is an organic acidaemia caused by a block in the catabolic pathway of isoleucine and valine (propionyl-CoA carboxylase). It usually presents in the first days of life with a marked metabolic acidosis with ketosis and raised lactate. The severity of the decompensation may switch off the bone marrow resulting in neutropenia, or even pancytopenia, and therefore may be confused with sepsis. Moderate hypocalcaemia is common. Hyperammonaemia may occur due to secondary impairment of the urea cycle. Normoglycaemia or hyperglycaemia are seen, rather than hypoglycaemia. Other acute complications include globus pallidus necrosis, cardiomyopathy and pancreatitis.

16. B: Glucose-6-phosphatase deficiency (GSD I)

These are all glycogen storage disorders (GSD). Hypoglycaemia is not a feature of the muscle GSDs V (phosphofructokinase) and GSD VII (myophosphorylase). Later onset of muscle fatigue and myalgia is their usual presentation. Branching enzyme deficiency produces long glycogen chains that act like amylopectin to produce cirrhosis and ultimately liver failure. Hypoglycaemia is a feature of the liver GSDs: GSD I (a or b), GSD III, GSD VI and GSD IX, although it is usually mild (or absent) in the last two conditions. The results of the investigations identify glucose-6–phosphatase deficiency as the cause. The biochemical signature of GSD I is hypoglycaemia, with raised lactate, urate and triglycerides. Hypoglycaemia occurs once the exogenous sources of glucose are exhausted as glycogenolysis and gluconeogenesis are blocked. Presentation may be delayed by many months as long as regular and frequent feeds are taken (eg prop-feeding or demand feeding overnight). Breakdown of glycogen to pyruvate is intact, however, and lactate is therefore produced as a secondary fuel for the brain. Conversion of lactate and pyruvate to fatty acids and cholesterol results in hyperlipidaemia. Uric acid production is increased from glucose-6-phosphate.

17. E: Diazoxide

Hypoketotic hypoglycaemia has a limited differential diagnosis, and the failure of rapid reversal following a bolus and the requirement of a continued dextrose infusion is suggestive of hyperinsulinism. The coexistence of hyperammonaemia suggests HIHA (hyperinsulinism hyperammonaemia) syndrome. This is due to upregulation of glutamate dehydrogenase. Diagnosis may be delayed by several months if the child has access to regular feeds, for example by continued breast or bottle feeding every few hours throughout the night and day. HIHA is exquisitely responsive to diazoxide to control the hyperinsulinism and it is the treatment of choice. The hyperammonaemia is controlled with mild-to-moderate dietary protein restriction.

18. A: Ammonia

The finding of a respiratory alkalosis in a sick neonate is an unusual finding and is not consistent with acidosis or a primary lung pathology causing the tachypnoea. Ammonia is a respiratory stimulant which acts directly on the brainstem and should be measured in any child with encephalopathy and a respiratory alkalosis.

19. C: Renal tubular acidosis

Metabolic acidosis in the presence of a normal anion gap indicates bicarbonate loss, rather than the presence of excess acids. The two potential routes for loss are the gut and kidney with the former less likely in the absence of loose stool. Renal tubular acidosis is therefore the most likely diagnosis. Inborn errors of metabolism are unlikely to be the cause of an acidosis in the absence of either a raised lactate or ketosis.

20. B: Maternal plasma amino acids

Excess phenylalanine is teratogenic. Uncontrolled maternal PKU can therefore damage the unborn child with common adverse features including growth retardation, microcephaly, mental retardation, and cardiac anomalies. The child will be a carrier for PKU – but is unlikely to have PKU – because the risk of the father being a carrier is 1 in 50 (unless he is related). Excluding maternal PKU as the cause requires plasma phenylalanine measurement in the mother. Urinary amino acids are unreliable as they only reflect renal threshold, and therefore it is possible to have levels sufficiently high in the blood to damage a fetus, but normal in the urine.

answers

21. B: Acylcarnitines

MCAD is suggested by the hypoketotic hypoglycaemia and dicarboxylic aciduria. Ketone production is severely limited as ketones are the ultimate product of the blocked fat oxidation pathway. Dicarboxylic acids are formed when fatty acids undergo Ω-oxidation in the microsomes. Intercurrent illness, especially involving vomiting and diarrhoea, is a common precipitant of decompensation. Diagnosis is made on plasma acylcarnitine analysis by an elevated octanoylcarnitine (C8) level. Diagnosis would then be confirmed on genotyping for the common *G985* mutation. Fibroblast studies are used to confirm long-chain fat oxidation defects and are not usually necessary in MCAD diagnosis.

22. E: Tay–Sachs disease

A cherry red spot is seen in Niemann–Pick type C (NPC), Tay–Sachs and Sandhoff disease, all of which may present with developmental delay and regression. Tay–Sachs is not associated with organomegaly, unlike NPC and Sandhoff disease. Hyperacusis may be noted as being startled by sound from an early age.

23. INVESTIGATIONS OF INBORN ERRORS

1.   A – Very long chain fatty acids
Zellweger syndrome is a disorder of peroxisomal biogenesis. Elevated very long chain fatty acids (VLCFAs) are indicative of peroxisomal disorders because very long chain fat oxidation occurs within peroxisomes.

2.   D – Plasma amino acids
MSUD is diagnosed by the elevation of the branched-chain amino acids (BCAAs) leucine, isoleucine, and valine. Plasma amino acids are preferred because urinary amino acids reflect the renal threshold, and therefore the abnormality will be first detected in the blood.

3.   G – Urate
Lesch–Nyhan syndrome is a disorder of purine metabolism. Urate is grossly elevated due to the block in purine salvage, resulting in increased purine synthesis. Urate measurement is a key initial investigation in purine disorders.

24. EYE SIGNS IN INBORN ERRORS

1.   E – Pigmentary retinopathy
Pigmentary retinopathy is associated with long chain hydroxy acyl-CoA dehydrogenase (LCHAD) deficiency. It develops with time despite good control. The underlying mechanism is still unclear.

2.   G – Cataract
Cataracts are usually present at birth in galactosaemia. The cataracts are transparent to begin with (oil drop cataracts) and are therefore easily missed because the red reflex is preserved. If the condition remains undiagnosed, the cataracts mature and become denser. The cataracts can completely resolve if a diet free from lactose and galactose is started early.

3. B – Corneal clouding
Corneal clouding is associated with all the mucopolysaccharidoses, with the exception of Hunter syndrome (MPS type II). The degree of clouding may be very subtle and only revealed on slit-lamp examination. Morquio syndrome (MPS type IV) is typified by severe skeletal involvement (dysostosis multiplex), with sparing of the central nervous system.

25. LIVER FAILURE

1. E – Galactosaemia
Galactosaemia classically presents towards the end of the first week. Milder forms may present at a few months of age with renal tubular acidosis secondary to proximal tubular damage. Hepatomegaly may be marked, even reaching as far as the right iliac fossa. Clotting is always prolonged and bruising on presentation common. Jaundice is present within the first days and deepens with time as liver function deteriorates. Cataracts are usually present from birth, but because of their initial transparent nature (oil drop) before they mature, they are easily missed as the red reflex is visible through them. If the diagnosis is missed they will become more obvious with time. If treatment is started early they will resolve completely. Sepsis is very common in galactosaemia at presentation, with special susceptibility to *E. coli*. Reducing substances in the urine may be positive in liver failure, no matter what the cause is, and has led to mis-diagnosis. Phenyllactate and 4–hydroxyphenyllactate are non-specifically raised in liver impairment, and the normal orotic acid rules out OTC as the cause (it does so in all three of these scenarios). The ammonia is slightly raised and is a non-specific finding in a sick infant, particularly with liver impairment (the liver being the home of the urea cycle). Fat oxidation defects can present with a Reye syndrome-like picture; however, one would expect hypoglycaemia to be a major feature.

2. C – Tyrosinaemia
This history would also be compatible with galactosaemia. However the presence of succinylacetone is pathognomonic for classical (type I) tyrosinaemia.

3. I – Hereditary fructose intolerance
The clue to the diagnosis of hereditary fructose intolerance is the timing of the presentation. Infants do not present prior to weaning when they are first exposed to fructose. Infants classically vomit and may prove very difficult to wean. If fructose exposure persists, hepatomegaly develops with deteriorating liver function and marked acidosis. Diagnosis is usually based on history and when fulminant liver failure has developed, genotyping is the safest way of securing the diagnosis because liver biopsy for enzymology is contraindicated due to the coagulopathy. Fructosuria is a benign disorder characterised by the excretion of fructose in the urine. Wilson disease is not a clinical entity in children under the age of 5 years.

Neonatology

Grenville Fox

Multiple Choice Questions

1. The following are recognised causes of seizures in the first week of life

- ○ A congenital myotonic dystrophy
- ○ B trisomy 21
- ○ C conjugated hyperbilirubinaemia
- ○ D non-ketotic hyperglycinaemia
- ○ E maple syrup urine disease

2. The following are associated with pulmonary hypoplasia

- ○ A autosomal recessive polycystic kidney disease
- ○ B unilateral renal agenesis
- ○ C rupture of membranes at 20 weeks' gestation
- ○ D tracheal atresia
- ○ E polyhydramnios

3. The risk of surfactant deficiency is increased in

- ○ A the second of twins
- ○ B maternal opiate use
- ○ C babies born at 38 weeks compared to 40 weeks
- ○ D meconium aspiration syndrome
- ○ E pulmonary haemorrhage

4. The following statements are true of reproductive function

- ○ A ovaries develop from the primitive gonad due to the influence of the X chromosome
- ○ B mullerian inhibition factor is produced by the testis
- ○ C the uterus and fallopian tubes develop in the absence of mullerian inhibition factor
- ○ D male pseudohermaphrodites have XX karyotype
- ○ E 21-hydroxylase deficiency causes female virilisation

questions

5. Congenital diaphragmatic hernia

○ A occurs most commonly due to failure of the retrosternal part of the septum transversum to form
○ B is more common on the left side
○ C is associated with karyotype abnormalities in approximately 60% of cases
○ D is associated with malrotation of the gut
○ E causes bilateral pulmonary hypoplasia

6. Neonatal listeriosis

○ A is caused by Gram-negative cocci
○ B is usually a nosocomial infection
○ C is associated with maternal contact with cats
○ D should be treated with third generation cephalosporins
○ E has a good outcome if treated with appropriate antibiotics

7. Polyhydramnios is associated with

○ A placental insufficiency
○ B pre-term birth
○ C cleft lip and palate
○ D Möbius syndrome
○ E duodenal atresia

8. Haemorrhagic disease of the newborn (vitamin K deficiency bleeding)

○ A is more common in formula-fed infants
○ B is more likely to occur in breast-fed infants if the mother is being treated with heparin
○ C usually presents with petechiae
○ D leads to prolongation of the activated partial thromboplastin time
○ E can be prevented by treating mothers with vitamin K supplements antenatally

9. The following are recognised causes of conjugated hyperbilirubinaemia in the newborn

○ A intrahepatic biliary hypoplasia
○ B polycythaemia
○ C galactosaemia
○ D tyrosinaemia
○ E β-thalassaemia

10. The following are risk factors for periventricular leucomalacia

○ A maternal opiate use
○ B maternal cocaine use
○ C chorioamnionitis
○ D antepartum haemorrhage
○ E hyperbilirubinaemia

11. Fetal haemoglobin

○ A consists of two α and two γ chains
○ B is approximately 80% of the total haemoglobin at term
○ C causes the oxyhaemoglobin dissociation curve to be shifted to the right
○ D is undetectable in adults
○ E is unaffected by sickle cell disease

12. The following increase the risk of vertical transmission of human immunodeficiency virus

○ A high maternal CD4 count
○ B twin pregnancy
○ C prolonged rupture of membranes
○ D pre-term birth
○ E Caesarian section

13. The following are recognised causes of symmetrical intrauterine growth restriction

○ A trisomy 18
○ B altitude
○ C maternal smoking
○ D fetal alcohol syndrome
○ E maternal antiphospholipid syndrome

14. The following is true of Erb's palsy

○ A the C8 to T1 nerve roots are usually involved
○ B the grasp reflex is usually preserved
○ C the Moro reflex is reduced
○ D denervation of the deltoid muscle occurs
○ E full recovery occurs in the majority of cases within 6 months

15. The following are recognised causes of hyperchloraemia in the newborn

○ A total parenteral nutrition
○ B treatment with loop diuretics
○ C fluid resuscitation with normal saline
○ D proximal renal tubular acidosis
○ E nephrogenic diabetes insipidus

16. The following are recognised causes of hypocalcaemia in the newborn

- ○ A maternal hypoparathyroidism
- ○ B maternal diabetes
- ○ C Di George syndrome
- ○ D hypermagnesaemia
- ○ E hypophosphataemia

17. The following statements about twin pregnancy are true

- ○ A twins with different blood groups are dizygous
- ○ B dichorionic twins are always dizygous
- ○ C dichorionic placentas always have two amnions
- ○ D assisted conception has led to a recent increased rate of monozygous twin pregnancy
- ○ E perinatal mortality is higher in dizygotic than in monozygotic twin pregnancy

18. The following statements about nutrition in the newborn are true

- ○ A energy requirements are higher in infants on parenteral nutrition than infants fed enterally
- ○ B the predominant protein of human milk is casein - whey
- ○ C approximately 50% of energy in human milk is fat-derived
- ○ D glucose is the predominant carbohydrate source in human milk
- ○ E the sodium content of human milk is inadequate for very-low-birthweight infants

Best of Five Questions

19. A baby is born by spontaneous, vaginal delivery at 35^{+6} weeks' gestation following rupture of membranes 30 hours before birth. The mother was well and not treated with antibiotics during labour. A vaginal swab was taken on admission. The baby was well and the mother wishes to be discharged home as soon as possible. The MOST appropriate course of action for the baby at this time is which of the following?

- A Discharge home
- B Observe in hospital for 48 hours
- C Await result of vaginal swab and treat the baby according to this
- D Perform an infection screen and treat with intravenous antibiotics if results suggestive of sepsis
- E Perform an infection screen and treat with intravenous antibiotics for at least 48 hours pending results

20. A well 3-week-old baby born at term is referred to hospital with a discharging umbilicus. The cord separated at 10 days and there is no peri-umbilical swelling or erythema. There is a small red mass at the site of cord separation, which is discharging a small amount of yellow fluid. The GP had taken a swab of this which grew *Staphylococcus epidermidis*. The MOST appropriate course of action is which of the following?

- A Reassure parents and review in 1–2 weeks
- B Treat with oral antibiotics
- C Treat with intravenous antibiotics
- D Arrange an abdominal ultrasound scan
- E Refer to a paediatric surgeon

21. A term baby presented with severe respiratory failure, which did not respond to initial resuscitative efforts, resulting in the baby's death at 20 minutes of age. Antenatal ultrasound scans had shown anhydramnios and large fetal kidneys with numerous large fluid-filled cysts. The liver appeared normal and no other anomalies were seen. Both parents had a normal renal ultrasound scan. What is the MOST likely diagnosis?

- A Autosomal recessive polycystic kidney disease
- B Autosomal dominant polycystic kidney disease
- C Posterior urethral valves
- D Bilateral multicystic dysplastic kidneys
- E Meckel–Gruber syndrome

22. **A well, breast-feeding term infant presented with jaundice at 36 hours of age. The serum bilirubin was 286 μmol/L, direct Coombs test negative, blood film showed spherocytes and reticulocytes, the baby's blood group was A rhesus negative and mother's blood group O Rhesus negative. Which of the following is the MOST likely diagnosis?**

- A Rhesus haemolytic disease
- B ABO incompatibility
- C Hereditary spherocytosis
- D Physiological jaundice
- E Breast milk-associated jaundice

23. **A woman develops chickenpox 2 days before giving birth to a healthy term baby. Which of the following is the treatment of choice?**

- A No treatment necessary for mother or baby
- B Treat mother with aciclovir
- C Treat mother with varicella zoster immune globulin only
- D Treat baby with varicella zoster immune globulin only
- E Treat baby with varicella zoster immune globulin and aciclovir if chickenpox develops

24. **A term baby born after spontaneous vaginal delivery is noted to be pale. Full blood count shows hemoglobin 5.4 g/dL; white cell count 15.1 × 10⁹/L; platelets 286 × 10⁹/L. The blood film is normal. The baby remains well and is transfused with packed red blood cells. A cranial ultrasound scan is normal. In order to establish the cause of the anaemia, the NEXT investigation should be which one of the following?**

- A Abdominal ultrasound scan
- B Coagulation screen
- C Apt's test
- D Kleihauer test
- E Bone marrow biopsy

25. **A girl infant has profound hypotonia and required intubation and positive pressure ventilation immediately after birth. She was born at term following a pregnancy complicated by polyhydramnios and reduced fetal movements. The chest X-ray shows small, but clear, lung fields. What is the MOST likely diagnosis?**

- A Trisomy 21
- B Neonatal encephalopathy
- C Congenital myotonic dystrophy

○ D Cervical spinal injury
○ E Spinal muscular atrophy

26. A 7-day-old term boy is admitted to hospital with bruising and bleeding from the umbilical stump. He had been born at home and was not given vitamin K after birth. The full blood count is normal, but prothrombin time and activated partial thromboplastin time are elevated. What is the BEST treatment for the baby?

○ A No treatment
○ B Intramuscular vitamin K only
○ C Intravenous vitamin K only
○ D Intravenous vitamin K plus fresh frozen plasma
○ E Intramuscular vitamin K plus fresh frozen plasma

27. A pre-term infant born at 25 weeks' gestation is now 36 weeks corrected gestational age and is screened for retinopathy of prematurity. Both eyes are found to have stage 2 retinopathy of prematurity. Which ONE of the following should you tell the parents about the baby?

○ A No further screening or treatment is required and the visual prognosis is good
○ B No further screening or treatment is required but spectacles are likely to be required later
○ C No further treatment is required at this stage but further screening is necessary and the visual prognosis is likely to be good
○ D Treatment is required with laser therapy or cryotherapy
○ E There are retinal detachments and visual prognosis is poor

Extended Matching Questions

28. Theme: Patterns of dysmorphology and congenital malformations

A   VACTERL association
B   CHARGE association
C   Trisomy 13
D   Trisomy 18
E   22q deletion
F   Noonan syndrome
G   Fetal alcohol syndrome
H   Goldenhar syndrome
I   Rubinstein–Taybi syndrome
J   Congenital rubella

For each of the following case scenarios select the most likely diagnosis from the list above. Each option may be used once, more than once, or not at all.

○   1. Term baby, birth weight 3.2 kg, facial dysmorphism with cleft lip and palate, heart murmur.

○   2. Term baby, birth weight 3.9 kg, facial asymmetry with abnormal left pinna. Hemivertebrae in cervical and thoracic spine. Heart murmur.

○   3. Baby born at 30 weeks, birth weight 700 g, microcephaly, complex congenital heart disease, congenital diaphragmatic hernia, facial dysmorphism, abnormal fingers.

29. Theme: Neonatal jaundice

A   Physiological jaundice
B   G6PD deficiency
C   ABO incompatibility
D   Crigler–Najjar syndrome
E   Congenital hypothyroidism
F   Hereditary spherocytosis
G   Rhesus incompatibility
H   Gilbert syndrome
I   Biliary atresia
J   Galactosaemia

For each of the following case scenarios select the most likely diagnosis from the list above. Each option may be used once, more than once, or not at all.

○   1. A term, boy baby presented at 5 days of age, unwell with jaundice, vomiting, poor feeding and hypotonia. Initial investigation results were as follows: total bilirubin 660 μmol/L (conjugated 18 μmol/L); baby's blood group O Rhesus negative; mother's blood group O Rhesus positive; direct Coombs test negative; haemoglobin 8.7 g/dL; blood film: reticulocytes ++; thyroid stimulating hormone 4.1 mU/L.

○ 2. A well, 4-day-old term baby girl presents with jaundice at 4 days of age. Initial investigation results were as follows: total bilirubin 310 μmol/L (conjugated 8 μmol/L); baby's blood group A Rhesus negative; mother's blood group O Rhesus positive; direct Coombs test negative; haemoglobin 14.7 g/dL; blood film: few spherocytes and reticulocytes; thyroid stimulating hormone 2.3 mU/L.

○ 3. A well 16-day-old girl, born at 35 weeks' gestation, is investigated for jaundice. Initial investigation results were as follows: total bilirubin 180 μmol/L (conjugated 6 μmol/L); baby's blood group O Rhesus positive; mother's blood group B rhesus positive; direct Coombs test negative; haemoglobin 13.5 g/dL; blood film: normal; thyroid stimulating hormone 4.9 mU/L.

30. Theme: Neonatal sepsis

A Flucloxacillin
B Vancomycin
C Amoxicillin
D Benzylpenicillin
E Gentamicin
F Erythromycin
G Pyrimethamine
H Cefotaxime
I Amoxicillin and gentamicin
J Benzylpenicillin and gentamicin

For each of the following cases select the most appropriate antibiotic or antibiotic combination from the list above. Each option may be used once, more than once, or not at all.

○ 1. A pre-term infant, unwell with increasing incidence of apnoea and bradycardia. Blood culture grows *Staphylococcus epidermidis*.

○ 2. A baby born at 34 weeks' gestation, following spontaneous rupture of membranes with discoloured amniotic fluid, in poor condition with a pustular rash.

○ 3. A 26-week gestation baby ventilated for chronic lung disease is investigated for increasing ventilatory requirement and increasing quantities of yellow secretions from the endotracheal tube. Culture of these grows *Chlamydia* spp.

answers

1. Seizures in the first week of life

Answers: D E

Congenital myotonic dystrophy typically presents with hypotonia and sometimes with respiratory failure. Trisomy 21 presents with typical dysmorphic features and hypotonia. Profound unconjugated hyperbilirubinaemia may cause kernicterus, of which seizures may be a feature, whereas conjugated hyperbilirubinaemia is not a cause of seizures. Non-ketotic hyperglycinaemia may present with increased fetal movements, which are actually in-utero seizures and neonatal encephalopathy presenting as hypotonia and seizures from birth. Maple syrup urine disease (MSUD), in its most severe form, presents as collapse with encephalopathy, including seizures, usually from the third day of life.

2. Pulmonary hypoplasia

Answers: A C E

Primary pulmonary hypoplasia is rare. Secondary hypoplasia may be due to decreased amniotic fluid volume during the second trimester, which is most commonly due to rupture of membranes prior to 24 weeks' gestation or decreased fetal urine production. Decreased fetal urine production results from bilateral renal disease, including bilateral renal agenesis ('classical' Potter syndrome), bilateral cystic dysplastic kidneys, polycystic kidney disease (usually autosomal recessive but rarely autosomal dominant) or obstructive uropathy affecting both kidneys (eg posterior urethral valves). Neuromuscular disease such as congenital myotonic dystrophy and congenital structural myopathies lead to polyhydramnios due to decreased swallowing and also pulmonary hypoplasia due to decreased fetal breathing movements which are essential for normal lung development. Tracheal atresia prevents fluid leaving the fetal airways and enhances lung growth. Fetal surgery with tracheal plugging has been used successfully to promote lung growth in congenital diaphragmatic hernia, which along with other thoracic space occupying lesions is also associated with pulmonary hypoplasia.

3. Surfactant deficiency

Answers: A C D E

The risk of surfactant deficiency is increased by prematurity, with an incidence of approximately 90% at 26 weeks' gestation, 55% at 32 weeks, 3% at 38 weeks and <1% at 40 weeks. The incidence and severity is reduced by maternal antenatal steroids (dexamethasone and betamethasone), maternal opiates, in females and small for gestational age babies. The incidence and severity is increased in males, sepsis, babies of mothers with diabetes, those delivered by elective Caesarian section and with a strong family history of surfactant deficiency. Meconium aspiration syndrome and pulmonary haemorrhage has been shown to inactivate the action of endogenous surfactant and exogenous surfactant therapy has been shown to improve outcome in both conditions.

4. Reproductive function

Answers: B C E

The *SRY* gene on the Y chromosome influences the primitive gonads to form testes. The testes 'secrete' Mullerian inhibition factor (MIF) which results in regression of the uterus and fallopian tubes. Male pseudohermaphrodites have male karyotype (XY) but are under-virilised, most commonly due to androgen insensitivity. The most common cause of female pseudohermaphroditism (XX karyotype) is congenital adrenal hyperplasia due to 21-hydroxylase deficiency, which leads to increased levels of 17α-hydroxyprogesterone.

5. Congenital diaphragmatic hernia

Answers: B D E

The Buchdalek type of congenital diaphragmatic hernia is the most common. This arises due to failure of closure of the posterolateral canals within the septum transversum. Rarer anterior or Morgagni diaphragmatic hernia arises when the retrosternal part of the septum transversum fails to form. Congenital diaphragmatic hernia is more common on the left side (approximately 85% of cases). Karyotype anomalies occur in approximately 30% of cases. Other congenital malformations include congenital heart disease and malrotation of the intestine.

6. Neonatal listeriosis

Answer: All false

Listeriosis is caused by the Gram-positive coccobacillus *Listeria monocytogenes*. Neonatal infection is usually acquired in utero after the mother has become infected from food, often from un pasteurised dairy products or paté. Maternal contact with farm animals is thought to be a risk factor also. *Listeria* is often resistant to cephalosporins and amoxicillin is the antibiotic treatment of choice. Outcome after neonatal listeriosis is variable with a significant mortality (approximately 10%) and risk of long-term neuro-disability.

answers

7. Polyhydramnios

Answers: B D E

Polyhydramnios may be caused by maternal diabetes, karyotype abnormalities, twin-to-twin transfusion syndrome (polyhydramnios oligohydramnios syndrome), neuromuscular disorders (congenital myotonic dystrophy, congenital myopathies, spinal muscular atrophy and Möbius syndrome), oesophageal atresia (and other high intestinal atresias) and congenital diaphragmatic hernia. Some cases, particularly mild polyhydramnios, may be unexplained.

8. Haemorrhagic disease of the newborn

Answers: D E

Haemorrhagic disease of the newborn is caused by vitamin K deficiency. Vitamin K crosses the placenta poorly and breast milk contains low levels. Maternal liver disease and anticonvulsants (phenytoin and phenobarbitone) increase the risk, which can be reduced by supplementing mothers with vitamin K antenatally. Early-onset haemorrhagic disease of the newborn presents within the first 48 hours, usually with gastrointestinal bleeding. Classic disease presents in the first week of life with bruising, bleeding from the umbilical stump, and gastrointestinal tract bleeding. Intracranial haemorrhage may also occur but this is more common in late-onset haemorrhagic disease of the newborn, which occurs up to 6 months of age. The prothrombin time and activated partial thromboplastin time are prolonged as both the intrinsic and extrinsic pathways are affected. Maternal heparin therapy does not contraindicate breast-feeding.

9. Conjugated hyperbilirubinaemia in the newborn

Answers: A C D

Causes of conjugated hyperbilirubinaemia in the newborn are:

- Cholestasis secondary to total parenteral nutrition
- Intrauterine infection (hepatitis B, toxoplasmosis, rubella, cytomegalovirus, herpes simplex, coxsackie virus, adenovirus, syphilis)
- Bacterial sepsis
- Severe haemolysis
- Biliary atresia
- Intrahepatic biliary hypoplasia
- Choledochal cyst
- Metabolic causes (α1-antitrypsin deficiency, galactosaemia, tyrosinaemia, Gaucher's disease and other storage diseases, Rotor syndrome, Dubin–Johnson syndrome)
- Cystic fibrosis.

10. Periventricular leucomalacia

Answers: B C D

Periventricular leucomalacia is caused by ischaemia or infarction, but inflammation may also be part of the pathophysiological process. Events leading to periventricular leucomalacia may be antenatal, perinatal, or postnatal, and include maternal trauma, maternal severe illness, antepartum haemorrhage, chorioamnionitis, cord prolapse, hypotension, severe hypoxia and hypocarbia due to hyperventilation. Maternal cocaine use and pre-term birth are other risk factors. Maternal opiate use is associated with symptoms of withdrawal in neonates but this is not a risk factor for periventricular leucomalacia or other intracranial pathology. Severe hyperbilirubinaemia may lead to kernicterus, which predominantly affects the basal ganglia and auditory pathways. It is not associated with periventricular leucomalacia.

11. Fetal haemoglobin

Answers: A B E

Fetal haemoglobin consists of two α and two γ chains, whereas adult haemoglobin has two α and two β chains. The γ chains cause fetal haemoglobin to have reduced binding to 2,3-diphosphoglycerate, which shifts the oxyhaemoglobin dissociation curve to the left. Fetal red blood cells therefore have a higher affinity for oxygen. Approximately 80% of haemoglobin is fetal haemoglobin at term. This falls to less than 10% by 1 year of age and to less than 1–2% in adults. Sickle cell disease is caused by a mutation resulting in a substitution of valine for glutamic acid on the β chain. Therefore fetal haemoglobin is unaffected by sickle cell disease.

12. Vertical transmission of human immunodeficiency virus

Answers: C D

Approximately one-third of vertically transmitted cases of human immunodeficiency virus are transmitted across the placenta and two-thirds during birth. The risk of vertical transmission is increased by low maternal CD4 count, high maternal viral load, presence of p24 antigen in the mother, rupture of membranes greater than 4 hours before birth, pre-term birth, vaginal delivery, and no maternal anti-retroviral treatment. With maternal anti-retroviral treatment during the third trimester and to the baby for the first 6 weeks of life, without these risk factors, vertical transmission can be reduced to less than 1–2%.

13. Intrauterine growth restriction

Answers: A D

Causes of symmetrical intrauterine growth restriction include chromosomal anomalies (typically trisomy 18), intrauterine infections (cytomegalovirus, toxoplasmosis, rubella) and fetal alcohol syndrome. Asymmetrical intrauterine

answers

growth restriction is usually due to placental insufficiency and is much more common. Maternal conditions such as hypertension, pre-eclampsia, lupus, antiphospholipid syndrome, maternal renal disease and opiate use are associated with symmetrical intrauterine growth restriction. The 'donor' twin in twin-to-twin transfusion syndrome is also at risk. Maternal smoking leads to a mean 10% reduction in birth weight. Babies of mothers living at high altitude also follow a similar pattern of asymmetrically reduced fetal growth.

14. Erb's palsy

Answers: B C D

Erb's palsy occurs as a result of peripartum brachial plexus injury in approximately 1 in 1000–2000 births. Risk factors include macrosomia, instrumental delivery and shoulder dystocia. The C5 and C6 nerve roots are most commonly damaged but, rarely, more extensive injury may involve nerve roots from C4 to T1. If C4 is involved, diaphragmatic palsy may occur, and if T1 is involved, the small muscles of the hand are affected, leading to loss of the grasp reflex. The Moro reflex is reduced on the affected side. Most cases of Erb's palsy have decreased abduction at the shoulder with internal rotation, decreased elbow flexion, and loss of wrist extension. Only about 20% fully recover, although there is usually adequate function of the affected arm. Recovery is rapid during the first 6 months but may continue until 18 months.

15. Hyperchloraemia in the newborn

Answers: A C D E

Total parenteral nutrition (TPN) may lead to hyperchloraemic acidosis in pre-term infants, which can be reduced by substituting the sodium chloride in TPN with sodium acetate. Use of normal saline for fluid resuscitation, flushes, and in arterial lines may also lead to hyperchloraemia and metabolic acidosis. Other causes of hyperchloraemia include proximal or distal renal tubular acidosis and nephrogenic diabetes insipidus. The latter may be inherited as an X-linked condition and leads to insensitivity of the distal renal tubule to antidiuretic hormone (ADH). This leads to polyuria with dilute urine which may cause polyhydramnios antenatally and dehydration postnatally, with raised plasma sodium, chloride and creatinine.

16. Hypocalcaemia in the newborn

Answers: B C

Early-onset neonatal hypocalcaemia occurs secondary to prematurity, maternal diabetes and birth depression. Late-onset (after 3–5 days) hypocalcaemia may be due to hypoparathyroidism (transient idiopathic or congenital, as in Di George syndrome, maternal hyperparathyroidism and hypomagnesaemia), vitamin D deficiency (maternal vitamin D deficiency, liver and renal disease), rapid postnatal growth, hyperphosphataemia (impairs conversion of vitamin D to active form), loop diuretics, alkalosis and hypoalbuminaemia.

17. Twin pregnancy

Answers: A C

Monozygotic twin pregnancy occurs due to single ovulation with subsequent splitting. Zygosity may be determined after birth according to the sex and blood group of the twins, which are the same in monozygous (identical) twins. Chorionicity can be determined antenatally by ultrasound examination of the placenta and membranes. Monochorionic placentas are only found in monozygous twins, but approximately 30% of monozygous twin pregnancies are dichorionic. Only 4% of monozygotic twin pregnancies are monochorionic monoamniotic. Dizygotic twins always have dichorionic, diamniotic placentas. Techniques of assisted conception have increased the incidence of dizygotic twin pregnancy, whereas the incidence of monozygotic twin pregnancy has remained almost constant over recent years. Perinatal mortality is almost three times higher in monozygotic pregnancy than in dizygotic twin pregnancy, due to the increased risk of twin-to-twin transfusion syndrome.

18. Nutrition in the newborn

Answers: C E

Enteral feeding requires energy, therefore infants on parenteral nutrition generally have lower energy requirements. Human milk is whey-predominant (whey to casein ratio of approximately 3 : 2) whereas cow's milk is casein-predominant (whey to casein ratio of approximately 1 : 4). This is important for the provision of essential amino acids. Energy provision in human milk is by fat (approximately 50%), carbohydrate, predominantly as lactose (approximately 40%), and protein (approximately 10%). Sodium requirement of pre-term infants is as high as 5–6 mmol/kg/day. Human milk contains 0.7 mmol/100 ml of sodium and additional supplements are therefore required.

19. E: Perform an infection screen and treat with intravenous antibiotics for at least 48 hours pending results

Risk factors for neonatal sepsis include rupture of membranes greater than 12–24 hours, intrapartum maternal pyrexia (> 38°C), fetal tachycardia, chorioamnionitis, pre-term birth and maternal colonisation with group B *Streptococcus*. In this case there are two risk factors: prolonged rupture of membranes, and pre-term birth. Each risk factor represents approximately 1–2% risk of infection to the baby. Ideally the mother should have received intra-partum antibiotics and, if given greater than 4 hours prior to birth, the baby could have been considered adequately treated in the absence of other risk factors. In the absence of this, most guidelines suggest investigating well babies for sepsis and treating if there are two or more risk factors.

answers

20. A: Reassure parents and review in 1–2 weeks

The most likely diagnosis is umbilical granuloma. This is much more common than other possibilities, such as patent urachus and patent omphalomesenteric duct, which may present with discharge of urine or meconium. Umbilical granulomas are usually red and may discharge serous fluid or pus. Treatment with antibiotics is only necessary if omphalitis is a possibility, with peri-umbilical erythema in an unwell baby. Normal skin flora, such as *Staphylococcus epidermidis*, do not require antibiotic treatment. Cauterisation with silver nitrate may be considered but most umbilical granulomata are self-resolving within a few weeks.

21. D: Bilateral multicystic dysplastic kidneys

The pathophysiology in this case is severe fetal renal dysfunction, from as early as the second trimester, leading to anuria and subsequent anhydramnios, resulting in severe pulmonary hypoplasia. All of the listed diagnoses may do this. Autosomal recessive (infantile) polycystic kidney disease usually leads to large echo-bright kidneys on antenatal ultrasound scan, rather than macrocysts, and congenital hepatic fibrosis may be found. Autosomal dominant (adult) polycystic kidney disease usually presents later in life but may rarely be a cause of microcystic changes within the fetal kidneys. Posterior urethral valves are associated with bladder and renal tract dilatation. Meckel–Gruber syndrome is another cause of fetal renal cysts, but other abnormalities including encephalocoele, polydactyly, cardiac disease and liver disease are also found on antenatal ultrasound scan.

22. B: ABO incompatibility

The bilirubin level at this age is too high for physiological or breast milk-associated jaundice, which both tend to present later. Rhesus haemolytic disease is not possible as the baby is rhesus negative. Spherocytes and reticulocytes are seen commonly on the blood film in ABO incompatibility. The direct Coombs test is sometimes negative in ABO incompatibility, reflecting a low concentration of antibody on red blood cells.

23. E: Treat baby with varicella-zoster immune globulin and aciclovir if chickenpox develops

Perinatal chickenpox is a serious and potentially life-threatening disease. Approximately 25% of babies will become infected if their mother develops chickenpox in the peri-partum period. Maternal chickenpox within 5 days of birth presents the greatest risk, as there is insufficient time for transplacental transmission of antibodies. Administration of varicella zoster immune globulin (VZIG) within 72 hours of exposure has been shown to prevent and attenuate chickenpox. Development of symptoms in the baby may be as early as 3 days after the onset of the maternal rash, but may be up to 16 days. Mortality of untreated cases of perinatal chickenpox has been reported to be as high as 30%, therefore treatment with aciclovir is recommended if signs of this develop.

24. D: Kleihauer test

The most likely diagnosis is fetomaternal bleed leading to anaemia. This can be acute or chronic. The Kleihauer (Kleihauer–Betke) test is on maternal blood and detects the presence of fetal red blood cells, thus confirming or refuting the diagnosis of a fetomaternal bleed. The Apt's test is used if there is gastrointestinal bleeding to distinguish between maternal and baby's blood as the cause of this.

25. C: Congenital myotonic dystrophy

All options may cause neonatal hypotonia. Reduced fetal movements and polyhydramnios (due to reduced fetal swallowing) suggest a severe neuromuscular disorder. The small lung fields and ventilatory requirement suggest pulmonary hypoplasia, which may be secondary to severe neuromuscular disorders, which have an early in-utero onset (due to reduced fetal breathing movements). This makes neonatal encephalopathy and cervical spine injury unlikely because both of these nearly always occur secondary to an insult close to the time of birth. Although cases of spinal muscular atrophy with fetal onset have been described, they are extremely rare. Congenital myotonic dystrophy is therefore the best answer.

26. D: Intravenous vitamin K plus fresh frozen plasma

The diagnosis is haemorrhagic disease of the newborn (vitamin K-deficiency bleeding). This usually presents with gastrointestinal bleeding, bleeding from the umbilical stump and bruising after 2–7 days. Breast-fed babies not receiving vitamin K prophylaxis after birth are most at risk. The prothrombin time is elevated, as is the activated partial thromboplastin time to a lesser extent. With active bleeding it is important to give intravenous vitamin K because this will correct the deficiency quicker than the intramuscular route. Fresh frozen plasma should also be given because even intravenous vitamin K does not correct the clotting times quickly enough.

27. C: No further treatment is required at this stage but further screening is necessary and the visual prognosis is likely to be good

The main risk factors for retinopathy of prematurity (ROP) are prematurity and hyperoxia. All pre-term infants born before 32 weeks' gestation and/or 1500 g birth weight should be screened from 6 weeks of age. Staging determines treatment and prognosis and reflects the degree of neovascularisation. ROP stages 1 and 2 usually regress but continued screening is required until vascularisation is complete. Visual prognosis is good but there is an increased risk of refractive errors and squint. Stage 3 ROP

answers

usually regresses but requires close observation until vascularisation is complete as treatment with laser or cryotherapy may be required. There is a high incidence of refractive errors and squint. ROP stages 4 and 5 involve sub-total and total retinal detachment, usually with poor visual prognosis.

28. PATTERNS OF DYSMORPHOLOGY AND CONGENITAL MALFORMATIONS

1.   C – Trisomy 13
Features of trisomy 13 include holoprosencephaly, scalp defects, microophthalmia, cleft lip and palate, polydactyly, renal abnormalities, and congenital heart disease.

2.   H – Goldenhar syndrome
Features of Goldenhar syndrome include facial asymmetry with abnormal ears, deafness, epibulbar dermoid cysts, vertebral abnormalities, and congenital heart disease.

3.   D – Trisomy 18
Features of trisomy 18 include symmetrical intrauterine growth restriction, facial dysmorphism, clinodactyly, nail hypoplasia, rockerbottom feet, congenital heart disease, diaphragmatic hernia, and renal abnormalities.

VACTERL association has the following features: vertebral abnormalities, anal atresia with or without fistula, cardiac malformations, tracheo-oesophageal fistula, renal abnormalities, and limb abnormalities. CHARGE association typically has the following features: colobomas, heart malformations, atresia of choanae, retardation of growth and development, genital hypoplasia in the male, and ear abnormalities. The 22q deletion (Di George or velocardiofacial syndrome) includes hypocalcaemia due to parathyroid gland hypoplasia, thymus hypoplasia (leading to increased susceptibility to infection due to T lymphocyte deficiency), congenital heart disease, and cleft palate. Noonan syndrome consists of facial dysmorphism (low-set ears, flat nasal bridge), a short webbed neck, and congenital heart disease (pulmonary valve stenosis and cardiomyopathy commonest).

The features of fetal alcohol syndrome include prenatal and postnatal growth failure, mid-face hypoplasia, flat nasal bridge, thin upper lip, microcephaly, and congenital heart disease. Rubinstein–Taybi syndrome consists of facial dysmorphism with hypertelorism and abnormal nose, with broad medially deviated thumbs and big toes, and microcephaly. In congenital rubella there is symmetrical intrauterine growth restriction, microphthalmia, cataracts, hepatosplenomegaly, and congenital heart disease.

29. NEONATAL JAUNDICE

1.   B – G6PD deficiency

The presenting signs suggest early kernicterus, made more likely by the extremely high unconjugated hyperbilirubinaemia. The low haemoglobin and presence of reticulocytes suggest severe haemolysis. This excludes Crigler–Najjar syndrome; and Gilbert syndrome only leads to mild unconjugated hyperbilirubinaemia. There are no apparent blood group incompatibilities, thus making G6PD deficiency the most likely diagnosis, which can be confirmed by biochemical assay.

2.   C – ABO incompatibility

There is a moderately elevated unconjugated bilirubin and a set-up for ABO incompatibility. The direct Coombs test may be positive or negative in ABO incompatibility and the blood film often shows spherocytes and reticulocytes.

3.   A – Physiological jaundice

Apart from the moderately raised unconjugated bilirubin, all investigations are normal. It is not unusual for pre-term infants to remain jaundiced for 3 weeks.

30. NEONATAL SEPSIS

1.   B – Vancomycin

Vancomycin is the antibiotic of choice for either methicillin-resistant *Staphylococcus aureus* (MRSA) or *Staphylococcus epidermidis* infection. Although some *S. epidermidis* is sensitive to flucloxacillin, treatment should start before sensitivities are available.

2.   I – Amoxicillin and gentamicin

Congenital listeriosis is a strong possibility as a diagnosis. *Listeria* is often not sensitive to cephalosporins. Amoxicillin may be more effective than benzyl-penicillin. To provide broad spectrum antibiotic cover until results of blood culture and sensitivity is available, gentamicin should also be given initially.

3.   F – Erythromycin

Intravenous erythromycin is the treatment of choice for *Chlamydia* pneumonia or conjunctivitis in the newborn.

Nephrology

Jim Hart and Chris Reid

Multiple Choice Questions

1. Complications of nephrotic syndrome include

- ○ A hyperlipidaemia
- ○ B malnutrition
- ○ C primary pneumococcal peritonitis
- ○ D prolonged bleeding
- ○ E pulmonary embolism

2. Features of glomerulonephritis include

- ○ A hypotension
- ○ B peripheral oedema
- ○ C haematuria
- ○ D hydronephrosis on ultrasound
- ○ E dysuria

3. The following is true of acute post-streptococcal glomerulonephritis

- ○ A it is the commonest cause of nephritis in children
- ○ B it is usual for C3 to remain low for many months after the initial nephritic illness
- ○ C it rarely occurs in children less than 5 years old
- ○ D hypertension, if present at presentation, is usually persistent
- ○ E the incidence of chronic renal insufficiency after acute post-streptococcal glomerulonephritis is less than 1%

4. With regard to immunoglobulin A (IgA) nephropathy

- ○ A the serum IgA is usually low
- ○ B it usually presents with recurrent macroscopic haematuria
- ○ C if it presents during childhood 40% develop end-stage renal failure
- ○ D angiotensin-converting enzyme (ACE) inhibitors are contraindicated
- ○ E it can be differentiated from Henoch–Schönlein purpura nephritis on the basis of the renal biopsy findings

questions

5. The following is true of proteinuria

- A it requires no further investigation if it occurs during an acute febrile illness
- B oliguria increases the degree of proteinuria on dipstick testing
- C urinary protein:creatinine ratio depends on how dilute or concentrated the urine is
- D children with orthostatic proteinuria require long-term follow-up
- E persistent proteinuria may precede chronic renal impairment in patients with renal disease

6. With regard to proximal renal tubular acidosis

- A it should be suspected when the urinary pH is < 5.3 in the face of systemic acidosis
- B urine pH can be acid (< pH 5.3)
- C it can be caused by galactosaemia
- D it can be caused by cystinuria
- E it can occur as part of Fanconi syndrome

7. The following is true of distal renal tubular acidosis

- A nephrocalcinosis is a recognised complication
- B there is impaired excretion of hydrogen ions
- C it is associated with hyperkalaemia
- D it can be secondary to obstructive uropathy
- E it can present with failure to thrive

8. The following is true of neonatal renal function

- A premature infants have the same glomerular filtration rate (in ml/kg/min/1.73m^2) as term infants
- B glomerular filtration rate increases by 50–100% during the first week of life in well term babies
- C nephrogenesis is complete by 36 weeks' gestation
- D fractional excretion of sodium (the ratio of excreted to filtered sodium expressed as a percentage) is commonly inappropriately high (> 1%) in very low birth weight infants
- E plasma bicarbonate is lower in newborns than in older children because the bicarbonate threshold is lower in newborns

9. The following suggest pre-renal, rather than intrinsic, renal failure

- A urea of > 15 mmol/L
- B urinary sodium < 10 mmol/L
- C urine output less than 1 ml/kg/hour
- D hypotension
- E urinary osmolality of > 500 mosmol/L

10. The following are associated with renal cysts

○ A nephronophthisis
○ B chronic renal failure
○ C tuberous sclerosis
○ D asphyxiating thoracic dystrophy
○ E renal dysplasia

11. The following is true of autosomal recessive polycystic kidney disease

○ A the gene for autosomal recessive polycystic kidney disease is found on chromosome 6
○ B large renal cysts (> 2 mm) on antenatal renal ultrasound scanning are characteristic
○ C it is always associated with some degree of hepatic fibrosis
○ D it is associated with cerebral aneurysms
○ E hypertension is an uncommon complication

12. The following is true of diuretics

○ A spironolactone exerts its potassium sparing effect by increasing potassium reabsorption in the proximal convoluted tubule
○ B loop diuretics cause hypokalaemia by increasing distal tubular sodium delivery
○ C thiazide diuretics act on antidiuretic hormone receptors in the collecting ducts
○ D loop diuretics can cause a metabolic alkalosis
○ E loop diuretics may potentially be nephrotoxic

13. The following is true of renal homeostasis

○ A in Conn syndrome renin levels are high
○ B in Conn syndrome excess aldosterone leads to hyperkalaemia
○ C renin increases blood pressure by converting angiotensin I to angiotensin II
○ D patients with renal artery stenosis typically have a hypokalaemic alkalosis
○ E typically patients with Addison's disease have hyperkalaemia and hyponatraemia

14. Characteristic features of Bartter syndrome include

○ A increased urinary chloride
○ B hypokalaemia
○ C hyperchloraemia
○ D metabolic acidosis
○ E recurrent episodes of dehydration

questions

15. The following is true of vesicoureteric reflux

- ◯ A inheritance is autosomal dominant
- ◯ B can be excluded on renal ultrasound
- ◯ C does not cause nephropathy after 5 years of age
- ◯ D 70% of grade II reflux will resolve by 5 years of age
- ◯ E it can be demonstrated using a MAG 3 renogram

16. The following are indications for dialysis in acute renal failure

- ◯ A creatinine of > 700 μmol/L
- ◯ B increasing hyperkalaemia not responsive to conservative treatment
- ◯ C hyperammonaemia
- ◯ D urine output less than 0.5 ml/kg/hour
- ◯ E metabolic acidosis not controllable with sodium bicarbonate

17. Nephrocalcinosis is a recognised complication of the following

- ◯ A William syndrome
- ◯ B steroids
- ◯ C prematurity
- ◯ D frusemide
- ◯ E captopril

18. Hypertension can present with

- ◯ A failure to thrive
- ◯ B VIIth cranial nerve palsy
- ◯ C petechiae
- ◯ D proteinuria
- ◯ E retinal haemorrhages

19. The following are recognised complications of chronic renal failure

- ◯ A hypercalcaemia
- ◯ B iron deficiency anaemia
- ◯ C secondary enuresis
- ◯ D delayed puberty
- ◯ E hypophosphataemia

20. Posterior urethral valves

- ◯ A are excluded by a normal renal ultrasound on day 1 of life
- ◯ B are rarely associated with chronic renal failure if corrected surgically immediately after birth
- ◯ C occur in both sexes
- ◯ D are associated with polyhydramnios
- ◯ E an intravenous urogram is the investigation of choice

21. Glomerular filtration rate

○ A is expressed as a function of weight in children
○ B is overestimated by creatinine clearance because of tubular reabsorption of creatinine
○ C can be measured with a radioisotope using blood sampling without the need for urine samples
○ D may be reduced by angiotensin converting enzyme inhibitors because they cause constriction of the efferent glomerular arteriole
○ E reaches the normal mature value during the second year of life

22. Diabetes insipidus

○ A is always associated with abnormally low levels of antidiuretic hormone
○ B is characterised by low plasma osmolality with inappropriately high urinary osmolality
○ C is associate with hyponatraemia
○ D is best treated initially by fluid restriction
○ E is a cause of polyhydramnios

Best of Five Questions

23. **A 7-year-old boy presents with a 10-day history of purpura on his arms and legs. He has had 3 days of pain and swelling of his ankles and left knee but is ambulant. On examination he is apyrexial, his capillary refill is 1 second, pulse 100 beats per minute, blood pressure 105/80 mmHg. Urine dipstick shows blood ++ and protein +++. Bloods on admission revealed haemoglobin 132 g/L, white count 6.7×10^9/L, platelets 273×10^9/L, sodium 140 mmol/L, potassium 3.7 mmol/L, urea 3.0 mmol/L, creatinine 42 μmol/L and C reactive protein < 2. Which of the following actions would be the BEST?**

- ○ A Commence intravenous cefotaxime
- ○ B Commence oral prednisolone
- ○ C Advise bed rest
- ○ D Measure his protein/creatinine ratio on early and morning urine for a week
- ○ E Measure his serum creatinine monthly for 6 months

24. **A 7-year-old presents with a 3-month history of severe intermittent left loin pain. There is no past medical history of urinary tract infection. On examination he is apyrexial, his blood pressure is 170/90 mmHg, pulse 90 beats per minute and he has a palpable renal mass on the left side. Urine dipstick is negative to blood and protein. Urine culture is negative. Renal ultrasound reveals significant left renal pelvis dilatation (anterio–posterior diameter 20 mm) with normal renal parenchyma and a normal right kidney and renal tract. Which is the MOST useful investigation to perform next?**

- ○ A Micturating cysto-urethrogram
- ○ B DMSA scan
- ○ C MAG-3 dynamic renogram
- ○ D Intravenous urogram
- ○ E Plain abdominal radiograph

25. A 5-year-old presents with a 2-day history of right-sided facial weakness. He has had headaches for 6 months. On examination he is drowsy. His blood pressure is 180/95 mmHg, pulse 100 beats per minute and he is apyrexial. He has a right-sided VIIth cranial nerve palsy and bilateral papillo-oedema. The rest of his cranial nerves are intact. Examination of his deep tendon reflexes reveals symmetrical hyper-reflexia in his lower limbs, with down-going plantars. He has a gallop rhythm, normal first and second heart sounds, an apex displaced to the mid-axillary line. There are no murmurs and no radiofemoral delay. Blood tests reveal the following: haemoglobin 83 g/L; white count 7.0 × 10⁹/L; platelets 293 × 10⁹/L; blood film: hypochromic normocytic anaemia only; C reactive protein < 2L; sodium 135 mmol/L; potassium 4.9 mmol/L; urea 11.5 mmol/L; creatinine 231 μmol/L; corrected calcium 1.79 mmol/L (2.2–2.7 mmol/L); phosphate 2.9 mmol/L (1.1–2 mmol/L); bilirubin 11 μmol/L (< 17 μmol/L); urine dipstick: protein + , blood not detected; renal ultrasound: 2 small kidneys with cortical thinning. The MOST likely underlying cause of these findings is which of the following?

- A Brain tumour
- B Coarctation of the aorta
- C Encephalitis
- D Haemolytic–uraemic syndrome
- E Reflux nephropathy

26. A 14-year-old girl presents with a 2-day history of painless macroscopic haematuria. There is no family history of renal or hearing problems. Physical examination is unremarkable. Blood pressure: 110/70 mmHg; temperature: 37° C; urine culture: no growth; renal ultrasound: normal; full blood count and clotting: normal; sodium 140 mmol/L; potassium 4 mmol/L; urea 5 mmol/L; creatinine 79 μmol/L; C3 and C4 levels normal. In clinic, 2 months later, the urine dipstick shows blood ++ and protein +. A hearing test is normal. What is the MOST likely diagnosis?

- A Alport syndrome
- B IgA nephropathy
- C Nephrolithiasis
- D Mesangiocapillary glomerulonephritis
- E Acute post-streptococcal glomerulonephritis

27. A 2-year-old boy presents with a history of chronic diarrhoea. His parents describe him as having a good appetite. On examination his weight is on the 0.4th centile and his height on the 25th centile. His blood pressure is 90/60 mmHg and pulse is 90 beats/min. Further examination is otherwise unremarkable. He is mildly dehydrated. Blood tests show: pH 7.47; pCO_2 5.3 kPa; pO_2 10 kPa; bicarbonate 30 mmol/L (normal range 20–28); urinary sodium 3 mmol/L; urinary chloride 4 mmol/L; serum sodium 135 mmol/L; potassium 2.7 mmol/L; Urea 3.2 mmol/L; creatinine 40 μmol/L; full blood count: normal; liver function tests: normal; plasma renin: raised. What is the MOST likely underlying diagnosis?

- A Bartter syndrome
- B Conn syndrome
- C Cystic fibrosis
- D Münchhausen by proxy by administration of diuretics
- E Renal artery stenosis

Extended Matching Questions

28. Theme: Renal syndromes

A   Acute post-streptococcal glomerulonephritis
B   Autosomal dominant polycystic kidney disease
C   Fanconi syndrome
D   Focal segmental glomerulosclerosis
E   Minimal change glomerulonephritis ╱
F   IgA nephropathy
G   Systemic lupus erythematosus (SLE) nephritis
H   Wilms' tumour

For each of the case scenarios select the most likely diagnosis from the list above. Each option may be used once, more than once, or not at all.

○ 1. A 2-year-old boy presents with a 3-week history of facial swelling. He has ankle and sacral oedema. Blood pressure is 90/60 mmHg. Urine dipstick shows protein +++, blood +. Sodium 130 mmol/L; potassium 3.5 mmol/L; urea 7.3 mmol/L; creatinine 60 μmol/L; albumin 15 g/dl; C3 and C4 levels are normal.

○ 2. A 15-year-old girl presents with 2-week history of facial swelling. She has generalised oedema. Blood pressure 170/80 mmHg. Urine dipstick shows protein +++, blood +++. Sodium 131 mmol/L; potassium 5.2 mmol/L; urea 10.3 mmol/L; creatinine 163 μmol/L; albumin 15 g/dl; anti-nuclear antibody screen negative; C3 level low; and C4 level normal. There is no remission of proteinuria after 5 weeks of prednisolone at 60 mg/m^2.

○ 3. A 10-year-old boy presents 2 weeks after a sore throat with painless haematuria. He has mild pre-tibial oedema. Urine dipstick shows protein ++, blood ++++. Blood pressure 170/100 mmHg. He is well perfused and has a gallop rhythm. Bloods show: sodium 130 mmol/L; potassium 6.5 mmol/L; urea 15 mmol/L; creatinine 230 μmol/L; albumin 25 g/dl; C3 level low, C4 level normal.

29. Theme: Tubular dysfunction

A Bartter syndrome
B Congenital toxoplasmosis
C Cystinosis
D Lowe syndrome
E Nephrogenic diabetes insipidus
F Insulin-dependent diabetes mellitus
G Reflux nephropathy
H Pseudohypoparathyroidism

For each of the following scenarios choose the most likely diagnosis from the list above. Each option may be used once, more than once, or not at all.

○ 1. A 6-month-old girl presents with recurrent episodes of dehydration. There is a history of polyhydramnios during the pregnancy. She is on the 0.4th centile for weight, the 10th centile for length, and she is clinically 10% dehydrated. Blood pressure is 80/60 mmHg. Investigations show: pH 7.47; pCO_2 4.5kPa; bicarbonate 32 mmol/L; sodium 135 mmol/L; potassium 2.1 mmol/L; chloride 80 mmol/L; urea 5 mmol/L; creatinine 52 μmol/L; serum renin raised; urinary sodium 40 mmol/L; urinary potassium 50 mmol/L.

○ 2. An 18-month-old boy presents with a 6-month history of polyuria and polydypsia. Examination reveals 2 cm hepatomegaly. He has swollen wrists and knees consistent with rickets. He is photophobic. Blood pressure 100/80 mmHg. Blood tests show: pH 7.25; pCO_2 3.5kPa; bicarbonate 18 mmol/L; sodium 130 mmol/L; potassium 2.7 mmol/L; Urea 7.2 mmol/L; creatinine 120 mmol/L; glucose 4.3 mmol/L; calcium 2.2 mmol/L; phosphate 0.7 mmol/L; alkaline phosphatase 2030 mmol/L; thyroid stimulating hormone (TSH) raised; thyroxine low; urine dipstick shows glycosuria and proteinuria + +; urine pH 6.2.

○ 3. A 2-year-old boy presents with failure to thrive. There is no history of vomiting or diarrhoea. He had cataracts detected in the neonatal period. He has global developmental delay and hypotonia. Investigations show: sodium 135 mmol/L; potassium 3.2 mmol/L; urea 3 mmol/L; creatinine 60 μmol/L; glucose 4.2 mmol/L; phosphate 1.5 mmol/L; corrected calcium 2.35 mmol/L; serum pH 7.29; bicarbonate 15 mmol/L; chloride 108 mmol/L; urine pH 5.5; urine dipstick glucose +.

30. Theme: Hyponatraemia

A   Chronic renal failure
B   Congenital adrenal hyperplasia
C   Craniopharyngioma
D   Cystic fibrosis
E   Diabetic ketoacidosis
F   Excessive intravenous administration of salt-poor fluid
G   SIADH (syndrome of inappropriate secretion of anti-diuretic hormone)
H   Urea cycle defect
I   Viral encephalitis

For each of the following scenarios choose the most likely cause of the child's condition from the list above. Each option may be used once, more than once, or not at all.

1. A 2-month-old boy presents with tachypnoea and poor feeding. He was born in good condition at 36 weeks' gestation by spontaneous vaginal delivery. On admission he weighed 5.0 kg. His respiratory rate was 80 breaths per min and he had marked intercostal recession. He was clinically diagnosed as having bronchiolitis and started on maintenance fluids of 0.18% sodium chloride and 4% dextrose at 31 ml/hour; 12 hours later he developed profound apnoeas requiring intubation and ventilation on intensive care. At this point he is well perfused and he is not oedematous. Investigations on admission to intensive care showed: serum sodium 115 mmol/L; serum potassium 4.2 mmol/L; serum urea 2 mmol/L; serum creatinine 41 μmol/L; serum pH 7.19; serum pCO_2 8 kPa; serum pO_2 8 kPa; serum bicarbonate 20 mmol/L; serum glucose 4 mmol/L; urine osmolality 400 mosmol; urine sodium 50 mmol/L; urine potassium 40 mmol/L.

2. A 2-week-old Caucasian boy presents with a 3-day history of poor feeding. He was born at term weighing 4.0 kg. On admission he weighs 3.6 kg, has dry mucous membranes and cool peripheries; temperature 37.5 °C; respiratory rate 60 breaths/min and pulse 170 beats/min. The rest of the examination is unremarkable. Initial investigations show: serum sodium 125 mmol/L; serum potassium 6.9 mmol/L; serum urea 6 mmol/L; serum creatinine 60 μmol/L; serum bicarbonate 18 mmol/L; serum glucose 2.7 mmol/L; serum haemoglobin 170 g/L; serum white cell count 18 × 10⁹/L; serum platelets 370 × 10⁹/L; serum C reactive protein (CRP) 5 mg/L; abdominal ultrasound: normal; urine sodium 50 mmol/L; urine microscopy: no white or red cells seen.

3. A previously healthy 5-year-old girl was admitted to hospital following a 4-day history of profuse vomiting and diarrhoea. There is no past medical history of note. She is tracking along the 5th centile for height and the 50th centile for weight. Her weight 1 month prior to admission was 16 kg. On admission she is lethargic, her capillary refill time is

6 sec, her temperature 38°C and pulse 160 beats/min, and she weighs 15 kg (9th centile). Initial tests show: serum pH 7.31; serum pCO_2 3.5kPa; serum bicarbonate 18 mmol/L; serum sodium 137 mmol/L; serum potassium 3.2 mmol/L; serum urea 6 mmol/L; serum creatinine 80 μmol/L; serum alanine aminotransferase 50 IU/L (normal 28–44); serum albumin 27 g/L (normal 30–45); serum glucose 3.8 mmol/L; urine sodium 4 mmol/L; urine potassium 102 mmol/L; urine osmolality 900 mosmol. She is given four 150-ml boluses of 0.18% sodium chloride 4% dextrose over the first 3 hours of resuscitation until she becomes well perfused. She is then started on maintenance fluids plus 10% correction over 24 hours (0.18% sodium chloride 4% dextrose with 20 mmol/L of potassium chloride at 120 ml/hour). After 12 hours she becomes drowsy, so she is re-examined. At this point her capillary refill is 1 sec, pulse 120 beats/min, blood pressure 130/70 mmHg, temperature 37°C. She then has a prolonged generalised seizure. Investigations at the time of the seizure show: serum sodium 115 mmol/L; serum potassium 4.2 mmol/L; serum urea 4 mmol/L; serum glucose 5 mmol/L; serum lactate 7 mmol/L; serum pH 7.2; serum base excess –7 mmol/L; serum pCO_2 6 kPa; urine osmolality 100 mosmol; urine sodium 20 mmol/L.

answers

1. Complications of nephrotic syndrome

Answers: A B C E

The mechanism of elevation of cholesterol and low-density lipoprotein (LDL) is unknown. Chronic proteinuria and steroid therapy can lead to muscle wasting, which can be masked by oedema. Loss of immunoglobulin in the urine and immunosuppression with steroids predisposes to infection, particularly pneumococcus. Loss of anti-thrombin III and protein C and protein S, dehydration with venous stasis, and increased blood viscosity cause an increased risk of thrombosis. Hypovolaemia due to shift of water from the intravascular to the interstitial space is common. Symptoms include abdominal pain and anorexia. If hypovolaemia is severe acute tubular necrosis can ensue.

2. Glomerulonephritis

Answers. B C

Any of the glomerulonephritidies can present with any of the renal syndromes: nephritic syndrome (hypertension, haematuria, renal impairment); nephrotic syndrome (oedema, hypoalbuminaemia, proteinuria); haematuria and/or proteinuria; or any combination of these. The renal syndromes are not specific for particular conditions and the same condition can present with different clinical features in different patients.

3. Acute post-streptococcal glomerulonephritis

Answers: A C E

Acute post-streptococcal glomerulonephritis typically presents 10–14 days after a streptococcal throat or skin infection with nephritic syndrome but can present with any of the renal syndromes described above. Hypertension due to oliguria and fluid overload is common at presentation. Persistent clinical abnormalities (hypertension, proteinuria and microscopic haematuria) occur in less than 5% of children followed up long term. C3 is low with a normal C4. Complement levels should be checked 3 months after the acute illness, because if C3 is persistently low this may indicate other glomerulonephritidies, such as systemic lupus erythematosus or mesangiocapillary glomerulonephritis.

4. IgA nephropathy

Answer: B

Serum IgA is normal. It can present with any of the renal syndromes. It is a cause of persistent microscopic haematuria without any other renal symptoms. It has a good prognosis with only 10% developing hypertension, proteinuria and renal impairment during childhood. ACE inhibitors can control hypertension and reduce proteinuria. Henoch–Schönlein purpura and IgA nephropathy are histologically indistinct and may be different spectrums of the same disorder.

5. Proteinuria

Answers: B E

Although proteinuria is common during acute febrile illnesses follow-up should be ensured to check the proteinuria resolves. Dipstick testing is a good screening test for proteinuria although there are pitfalls. The gold standard for quantification of proteinuria is measurement on a 24-hour urine collection; however, this is difficult to do in children. Estimation of protein:creatinine ratio on an early morning urine is a worthwhile compromise. Orthostatic proteinuria is a benign condition and does not usually require renal biopsy. In orthostatic proteinuria, proteinuria is absent when the patient is recumbent. Regardless of how dilute or concentrated a urine sample is, if the concentration of the substance being measured in the urine is factored by the concentration of creatinine in the urine, then the effect of alterations in urine concentration is eliminated.

6. Proximal renal tubular acidosis

Answers: B C E

Renal tubular acidosis should be suspected when there is alkali urine (pH > 5.8) in the presence of systemic acidosis and a normal anion gap. In proximal renal tubular acidosis there is failure to reabsorb bicarbonate. However, distal tubular hydrogen ion secretion is normal, so if plasma bicarbonate falls to low levels (16 mmol/L) acid urine can be produced. In distal renal tubular acidosis, hydrogen ion excretion is impaired so there is never acid urine. Proximal renal tubular acidosis can be part of Fanconi syndrome, of which there are a number of causes: cystinosis; tyrosinaemia; galactosaemia; Lowe syndrome; Wilson's disease; heavy metal poisoning; idiopathic. Cystinuria causes increased urinary excretion of cysteine leading to nephrolithiasis and it is distinct from cystinosis.

7. Distal renal tubular acidosis

Answers: A B D E

Distal – and very rarely proximal – renal tubular acidosis is a cause of nephrocalcinosis. Distal renal tubular acidosis can be primary isolated or secondary to obstructive uropathy, amphotericin or cyclosporin. Hypokalaemia is a feature, rather than hyperkalaemia, due to increased urinary losses.

8. Neonatal renal function

Answers: B C D E

At 36 weeks' gestation nephrogenesis is complete. However, glomerular filtration rate (ml/kg/min/1.73m^2) is less than 5% of adult values. Glomerular filtration rate rises with age and reaches adult values by age 2 years. The glomerular filtration rate of premature infants is markedly less than term infants, hence their susceptibility to renal impairment. The ability to reabsorb filtered sodium and conserve sodium in a salt- or water-depleted state is impaired in babies. Older children and adults who are salt-depleted have a urinary sodium of less than 10 mmol/L and a fractional excretion of sodium of less than 1%, whereas premature infants tend to have inappropriately high urinary sodium concentration in this state. Water concentrating ability is not mature until 2 years of age. The plasma bicarbonate concentration at which filtered bicarbonate appears in the urine (bicarbonate threshold) is low in the newborn (19–21 mmol/l), increasing to mature values of 24–26 mmol/l by 4 years.

9. Pre-renal renal failure

Answers: B D E

In pre-renal failure the kidney tries to conserve water and sodium, hence urinary sodium is low (< 10 mmol/L). During intrinsic renal failure urine concentrating ability is impaired so urinary osmolality is usually < 300 mosmol/L. Urea increases in renal failure of both types, haemoconcentration and during starvation so it is an unreliable measure of dehydration. Oliguria (< 2 ml/kg/h in a baby and < 1 ml/kg/h in an older child) could be due to either reason. A raised blood pressure, gallop rhythm, raised jugular venous pressure/pulse (JVP) and good peripheral perfusion suggest intravascular overload associated with intrinsic renal failure. Low blood pressure and poor capillary refill suggest a pre-renal cause.

10. Renal cysts

Answer: All true

Renal cysts found coincidentally on ultrasound scanning should not be dismissed. Nephronophthisis is a rare condition but the commonest genetic cause of chronic renal failure in children. It usually presents with gradual onset of polyuria and anaemia before progressing to end-stage renal failure (average age of end-stage renal failure is 13 years). Around 80% of children receiving prolonged haemodialysis for whatever cause have multiple renal cysts. Renal cysts are one of the diagnostic criteria for tuberous sclerosis. Patients with tuberous sclerosis may also have renal angiomyolipomas. Patients with cystic fibrosis may develop interstitial nephritis as a result of an allergic reaction to drugs or infection. They may also develop acute tubular necrosis as a result of nephrotoxic drugs such as gentamicin.

11. Autosomal recessive polycystic kidney disease

Answers: A C

Large echo bright kidneys, with or without cysts that are small (< 2 mm) are characteristic of autosomal recessive kidney disease. The severity of hepatic fibrosis varies from sub-clinical to overt liver disease, which is the dominant clinical feature. There are two gene loci for autosomal dominant polycystic kidney disease, the commonest of which is on chromosome 16, adjacent to the tuberous sclerosis gene. Autosomal dominant polycystic kidney disease is associated with cerebral aneurysms, subarachnoid haemorrhage, mitral valve prolapse, and hepatic cysts. Hypertension is a major clinical feature and it may be very difficult to treat.

12. Diuretics

Answers: B D E

Spironolactone blocks aldosterone-sensitive channels in the collecting ducts, which reabsorb sodium in exchange for potassium and hydrogen ions. Loop diuretics block the N–K–2Cl transporter in the loop of Henle, increasing sodium and chloride delivery to the distal convoluted tubule. Sodium is then re-absorbed in exchange for potassium and hydrogen ions resulting in a hypokalaemic metabolic alkalosis. Potassium secretion is proportional to distal tubular urine flow, distal tubular sodium delivery and aldosterone level. Thiazide diuretics block the sodium potassium co-transporter in the early distal convoluted tubule.

13. Renal homeostasis

Answers: D E

In Conn syndrome there is primary hyperaldosteronism. High aldosterone leads to extracellular fluid expansion, hypertension, hypokalaemia, alkalosis and renin suppression. Renin is produced by the juxtaglomerular apparatus in response to reduced renal perfusion (shock, renal artery stenosis and renal scars). Renin converts angiotensinogen into angiotensin I. Angiotensin-converting enzyme (ACE) converts angiotensin I to angiotensin II. Angiotensin II increases blood pressure by causing vasoconstriction and increasing aldosterone secretion from the adrenals. In Addison's there is aldosterone deficiency.

14. Bartter syndrome

Answers: A B E

This inborn defect in the Na–Cl–2Cl co-transporter in the loop of Henle results in urinary sodium, chloride and water loss. It is autosomal recessively inherited. Markedly increased urinary chloride and sodium with normal serum creatinine are typical. Increased delivery of sodium to the distal convoluted tubule result in reabsorption of sodium in exchange for potassium and hydrogen ions, resulting in metabolic alkalosis.

15. Vesicoureteric reflux

Answers: A D E

Vesicoureteric reflux (VUR) is 20–50 times more common in children with a family history of VUR. Grade I or II reflux cannot be excluded on ultrasound. The investigation of choice is micturating cysto-urethrogram. Reflux nephropathy can occur at any age, especially if there is associated detrusor dysfunction, as in patients with spina bifida. Vesicoureteric reflux predisposes to urinary tract infection.

A MAG 3 renogram can be used to demonstrate VUR by scanning over the kidneys while the child voids after all the isotope has drained from the upper tracts into the bladder. For this test to be reliable the child must be old enough to have bladder control and to void on command.

16. Dialysis in acute renal failure

Answers: B C E

Creatinine itself is not toxic and takes days to rise, even when there is no renal function, so there is no absolute level at which acute dialysis is indicated. Haemodialysis can aid removal of low molecular weight toxins, such as ammonia or salicylate. Acute renal failure results in impaired excretion of hydrogen and potassium ions. Hyperkalaemia can result in ventricular tachycardia and ventricular fibrillation. Oliguria is not in itself an indication for dialysis, however volume overload and resultant hypertension unresponsive to diuretics are. Acidosis may be refractory to sodium bicarbonate. Side effects of sodium bicarbonate are hypernatraemia and hypertension.

17. Nephrocalcinosis

Answers: A B C D

Nephrocalcinosis is usually part of a metabolic disorder. Nephrocalcinosis is common in distal renal tubular acidosis but rare in proximal renal tubular acidosis. Hypercalciuria can cause nephrocalcinosis. Hyperparathyroidism, vitamin D intoxication, Bartter syndrome, William syndrome, corticosteroids and frusemide cause hypercalciuria. At follow up, 27% of infants born at less than 32 weeks and 62% of infants with chronic lung disease have nephrocalcinosis. Low birth weight, diuretic therapy, inadequate dietary phosphate, and duration of oxygen therapy are risk factors.

18. Hypertension

Answers: A B D E

The decision to treat hypertension is determined by the level of blood pressure and the presence of end-organ damage. Hypertensive encephalopathy may cause headache, irritability, seizures and hyper-reflexia. Findings in hypertensive retinopathy include cotton-wool spots and flame-shaped haemorrhages. Only rarely will there be retinal or macular oedema. Hypertension can cause renal impairment, left ventricular enlargement, and heart failure.

19. Complications of chronic renal failure

Answers: B C D

The main causes of chronic renal failure in childhood are renal dysplasia, reflux nephropathy, glomerulonephritis, genetically inherited diseases, such as Alport syndrome or nephronophthisis and systemic diseases, such as systemic lupus erythematosus (SLE) and Henoch–Schönlein purpura (HSP). Phosphate retention leads to hypocalcaemia and secondary hyperparathyroidism and bone resorption. Reduced synthesis of 1,25 hydroxy-vitamin D_3 contributes to hypocalcaemia and leads to rickets. Anaemia is secondary to dietary iron deficiency, reduced red blood cell survival, and erythropoietin deficiency. Polyuria is usual until glomerular filtration rate falls to end-stage renal failure levels (less than 10 ml/min/1.73m²).

20. Posterior urethral valves

Answer: All false

A normal ultrasound on day 1 of life does not exclude posterior urethral valves because hydronephrosis may not be apparent until urinary flow has been established. Posterior urethral valves are always associated with some degree of renal dysplasia and around 25% will end up with chronic renal failure or end-stage renal failure. Renal dysplasia is known to occur even if the valves are operated on in utero. The classic presentation is of oliguria and pulmonary hypoplasia. They are associated with maternal oligohydramnios. They are best diagnosed on micturating cysto-urethrogram. To visualise the valves, films must be taken without the urinary catheter in situ.

21. Glomerular filtration rate

Answers: C E

GFR is expressed as a function of surface area (SA). Absolute values for GFR in ml/min are corrected for SA by the formula: Corrected GFR (ml/min/1.73m²) = absolute GFR (ml/min) x 1.73/SA (where 1.73m² is the SA of an average adult male). Creatinine clearance overestimates GFR because there is tubular secretion of creatinine. The standard way of measuring GFR involves the single injection plasma disappearance curve method, where inulin, or an isotope like ⁵¹-chromium labelled EDTA, is injected and serial blood samples are taken to allow a plot of the rate of clearance of inulin or the isotope from the plasma. Urine samples are not needed. ACE inhibitors cause dilatation of the efferent glomerular arteriole, thus lowering the hydrostatic pressure in the glomerular capillary bed, and hence the GFR may be lowered. The normal mature GFR value of 80–120 ml/min/1.73m² is reached during the second year.

22. Diabetes insipidus

Answer: E

Diabetes insipidus may be central due to reduced secretion of ADH when plasma levels will be low, or peripheral due to end organ resistance of ADH when plasma levels are usually around or just above the top end of normal range. The fundamental diagnostic feature is raised plasma osmolality with inappropriately low urine osmolality. With complete absence of action of ADH humans may produce urine osmolality of <100mOsm/L. Patients with diabetes insipidus commonly have urine osmolality higher than this, because there is not complete failure of secretion or complete end-organ resistance, but in comparison to the raised plasma osmolality the urine osmolality is still inappropriately low. Hypernatraemia is the characterisitic plasma electrolyte change. Treatment of acute hypernatraemic dehydration includes replacement of water deficit with extra intravenous fluid. However many patients manage to avoid these episodes as long as they have free access to water when they feel thirsty. The diagnosis is sometimes made when a patient is unable to have normal free access to fluid eg after routine surgery when nil by mouth, when they develop hypernatraemic dehydration despite what would normally be adequate IV replacement fluid.

Best of five

23. D: Measure protein/creatinine ratio on early-morning urine for a week

The scenario suggests Henoch–Schönlein purpura (HSP). Around 70% of children with HSP have some degree of renal involvement, usually just microscopic haematuria with or without mild proteinuria. Patients can develop nephritic syndrome, nephrotic syndrome, hypertension, or chronic renal failure, sometimes years after the original rash. Persistent nephrotic range proteinuria (protein/creatinine ratio > 200mg/mmol) warrants referral to a nephrologist for consideration of a biopsy. Arthritis usually settles without treatment. Bed rest does not alter the course of the condition. Serum creatinine is an insensitive measure of renal involvement, although it is of concern if raised. Steroids are rarely used in HSP but have been used for severe abdominal pain and severe glomerulonephritis.

24. C: MAG-3 dynamic renogram

The patient is most likely to have pelvi–ureteric junction obstruction from the scenario presented. The investigation of choice is a MAG-3 (dynamic renogram) to determine if there is obstruction to urinary flow. The patient is hypertensive (95th centile for systolic BP is 106+ [age × 2]). Hypertension of renal origin can occur by a number of mechanisms. It can occur when there is obstruction to urinary flow, as in this case. It can also occur because of reduced renal blood flow, either generally (as in renal artery stenosis) or locally (which occurs in renal scarring). Vesicoureteric flux with renal scarring from previous urinary tract infection is also a possibility, so DMSA and micturating cysto-urethrogram should be considered. However, vesicoureteric reflux without urinary tract infection would not cause loin pain. Abdominal X-ray and intravenous urogram would be indicated if nephrolithiasis were thought to be the cause of his pain. Nephrolithiasis is rare in childhood and in the absence of microscopic haematuria.

25. E: Reflux nephropathy

VIIth nerve palsy is a recognised complication of hypertension in childhood. The child presents with symptoms consistent with hypertensive encephalopathy, such as drowsiness, papilloedema and hyper-reflexia. The anaemia, low calcium, proteinuria, and high urea, creatinine and phosphate are consistent with chronic renal impairment. Renal impairment can cause hypertension, or be as a result of hypertension. The cardiovascular signs are consistent with heart failure, which could be as a result of hypertension. The absence of murmurs and radiofemoral delay makes coarctation less likely. Raised intracranial pressure could cause hypertension but would not explain the other findings. Recurrent urinary tract infections and vesicoureteric reflux are thought to cause renal scarring and reflux nephropathy.

Sometimes there is no history of urinary tract infection. This may be because the urinary tract infections have gone undiagnosed or because the renal abnormalities are congenital dysplastic renal malformations, which are indistinguishable from renal scars on DMSA and ultrasound scanning. Children with renal scars should have yearly blood pressure checks for life.

26. B: IgA nephropathy

IgA nephropathy can present as an incidental finding of persistent microscopic haematuria or with any of the renal syndromes. Prognosis is good although 10% will develop hypertension, proteinuria +/– renal failure with long-term follow-up. Alport syndrome, a hereditary nephritis, could present with a similar clinical picture. There are X-linked and autosomal recessive forms. Deafness around the age of 10 years, hypertension in mid-teenage years, and end-stage renal failure in the third decade is usual. Family members of children presenting with haematuria should be screened for microscopic haematuria and proteinuria. Nephronophthisis usually presents with polyuria/polydypsia, often has normal urinalysis and progresses to end-stage renal failure in the first decade. Acute post-streptococcal glomerulonephritis and mesangiocapillary glomerulonephritis could present in a similar way, however C3 is usually reduced. Typically, mesangiocapillary glomerulonephritis has persistently low C3, nephrotic range proteinuria (protein/creatinine ratio > 200mg/mmol), hypertension and progressive renal impairment.

27. C: Cystic fibrosis

The patient has a metabolic alkalosis with a very low serum potassium, the causes of which are: Bartter syndrome; pseudo-Bartter syndrome; aldosterone excess; renin excess; or diuretics. Pseudo-Bartter syndrome occurs when sodium and chloride are lost from extra-renal sites leading to a secondary hyper-reninaemia. Causes include cystic fibrosis, congenital chloride diarrhoea, laxative abuse and cyclical vomiting. The serum biochemistry is the same as Bartter syndrome (hypochloraemic, hypokalaemic alkalosis) but there are appropriately low levels of urinary chloride and sodium (< 10 mmol/L). Renin is released from the juxtaglomerular apparatus in response to reduced renal perfusion, leading to increased angiotensin II, which causes vasoconstriction and aldosterone release from the adrenals. Aldosterone causes extracellular fluid expansion by distal tubular sodium and water conservation. Sodium is reabsorbed in exchange for hydrogen ions and potassium. Hyper-reninaemic states, such as renal artery stenosis, can produce a similar biochemical picture to the scenario, however the patient is not hypertensive. Conn syndrome, primary hyperaldosteronism, also causes hypertension but there is renin suppression. Loop diuretics can produce a similar biochemical picture to the scenario, although there would be a high urinary sodium.

28. RENAL SYNDROMES

1. E – Minimal change glomerulonephritis

85% of toddlers presenting with nephrotic syndrome will have minimal change disease. This is usually steroid sensitive, renal function is normal, hypertension not sustained and microscopic haematuria mild and intermittent.

2. D – Focal segmental glomerulosclerosis

Steroid-resistant nephrotic syndrome is defined as no remission after 4 weeks of 60 mg/m^2 prednisolone. The usual histology is focal segmental glomerulosclerosis or membranoproliferative glomerulonephritis. The age of presentation is typically greater than 8 years or less than 1 year. The long-term prognosis is poor. Hypertension and microscopic haematuria are common.

3. A – Acute post-streptococcal glomerulonephritis

This child has nephritic syndrome (renal impairment and oliguria leading to hypertension and fluid overload). Many glomerulonephritidies can present with nephritic syndrome but it is reasonable to assume that the cause is acute post-streptococcal glomerulonephritis and not perform a renal biopsy if there is complete recovery of renal function and C3 levels return to normal after 3 months.

29. TUBULAR DYSFUNCTION

1. A – Bartter syndrome

The metabolic alkalosis and very low potassium suggests Bartter syndrome. This is due to an inborn defect in the N–K–2Cl transporter in the thick loop of Henle, leading to salt and water wasting. The resultant extracellular fluid (ECF) volume contraction leads to secondary hyperaldosteronism and avid sodium and water reabsorption in the distal convoluted tubule, and reciprocal potassium and hydrogen ion excretion into the urine. Crucial to the diagnosis is the finding of inappropriately high levels of urinary chloride and sodium.

2. C – Cystinosis

In this scenario there is glycosuria with normal serum glucose and metabolic acidosis with an inappropriately alkaline urine. This suggests there is a proximal tubular leak consistent with Fanconi syndrome. There are a number of causes of Fanconi syndrome such as galactosaemia, mitochondrial disorders, tyrosinaemia, fructosaemia, Lowe syndrome, Wilson's disease, cystinosis, and heavy metal poisoning. Cystinosis is an autosomal recessive defect in the transport out of lysosomes. It leads to a multisystem disorder. Early features include Fanconi syndrome, photophobia due to cysteine crystals in the cornea, and hypothyroidism. Renal failure occurs around 10 years of age if untreated. Diagnosis is confirmed by raised peripheral blood white cell cysteine levels.

3. D – Lowe syndrome

The occulocerebrorenal syndrome of Lowe is an X-linked disorder characterised by congenital cataracts, hypotonia, intellectual impairment, and renal Fanconi syndrome. Hypokalaemia is not marked. There is no specific treatment. Patients develop chronic renal failure in the second to fourth decades.

30. THEME: HYPONATRAEMIA

1. G – SIADH (syndrome of inappropriate secretion of anti-diuretic hormone) secondary to bronchiolitis

The apnoeas are likely to be due to hyponatraemic seizures rather than impending respiratory failure. This patient has inappropriately concentrated urine in the face of very dilute plasma (239 mosmol). The plasma osmolality is is given by:

$$2 \times (Na + K) + (urea + glucose)$$

The normal range is 275–295 mmol/L. To diagnose SIADH there must be evidence of fluid overload as well as signs of volume depletion. As water distributes freely between the ECF and ICF oedema is not usually present. In SIADH an increase in ECF volume and reduction in plasma osmolality fails to suppress anti-diuretic hormone (ADH) secretion and, if normal fluid intake is maintained, hyponatraemia develops. It is caused by surgery, or by pulmonary disorders, such as infections or positive pressure ventilation, or by disorders of the central nervous system, such as meningitis or hypoxic–ischaemic encephalopathy. Treatment is to restrict water intake.

2. B – Congenital adrenal hyperplasia

The inappropriately high urinary sodium in the face of hyponatraemia and hypovolaemia suggests an inability to reabsorb filtered sodium, broadly the causes of which are renal failure, aldosterone deficiency, and administration of diuretics. The relatively normal serum creatinine makes renal failure unlikely, although creatinine takes hours to rise in acute renal failure. With the exception of spironolactone most diuretics cause hypokalaemia. The combination of low sodium and glucose and high potassium suggests adrenal insufficiency, the causes of which are primary (such as congenital adrenal hyperplasia or Addison's disease) or secondary (such as panhypopituitarism or tumours affecting the pituitary, eg craniopharyngioma). The lack of cortisol and aldosterone in congenital adrenal hyperplasia leads to production of adrenocorticotrophic hormone (ACTH). ACTH acts on melanocyte-stimulating hormone receptors to cause pigmentation in skin folds. There are a number of forms of congenital adrenal hyperplasia, which can present at various ages in various ways. In classical congenital adrenal hyperplasia there is deficiency of one of the enzymes in the biosynthetic pathway of the adrenal cortex (21-hydroxylase deficiency). The continuing ACTH drive leads to the precursors being directed along the androgen biosynthetic pathway, causing virilisation. This presents with ambiguous genitalia in girls and a salt-losing crisis or precocious puberty in boys. Investigation involves karyotyping, serum 17-hydroxyprogesterone (the precursor of 21-hydroxylase), urinary steroid profile, and adrenal androgen levels. Acute treatment is with hydrocortisone and salt replacement.

3. F – Excessive intravenous administration of salt-poor fluid

The initial history and investigations are consistent with gastroenteritis with 10% dehydration. Although serum sodium is normal there will be a total body sodium deficit, as diarrhoea and vomit contain large amounts of sodium (75 mmol/L). The slightly low initial potassium indicates that the distal tubule is reabsorbing sodium at the expense of potassium. The girl is resuscitated with the equivalent of half her circulating blood volume (40 ml/kg) of salt-poor fluid and she then receives further salt-poor maintenance fluid. This will correct her water deficit but not the salt deficit, resulting in dilutional hyponatraemia.

Neurology

Tammy Hedderly

Multiple Choice Questions

1. In neurofibromatosis type 1

- ○ A 25% of cases have no previous family history of neurofibromatosis
- ○ B bony dysplasia is a diagnostic criterion
- ○ C brain magnetic resonance imaging is a routine diagnostic test
- ○ D there is a 10% risk of malignant change in plexiform neurofibromas
- ○ E optic gliomas occur predominately in children over 7 years

2. Friedreich's ataxia

- ○ A is caused by an expansion of GAA trinucleotide repeat
- ○ B motor nerve conduction velocities are usually normal
- ○ C usually presents in the first 6 years of life
- ○ D cardiomyopathy is the commonest cause of death
- ○ E requires pes cavus for the diagnosis

3. The following conditions are correctly paired with expected cerebrospinal fluid findings

- ○ A acute disseminated encephalomyelitis and CSF lymphocytosis with increased protein
- ○ B tuberculous meningitis and high glucose with raised protein
- ○ C Guillain Barré syndrome and normal cell count with reduced protein
- ○ D fungal meningitis and lymphocytic CSF with low glucose
- ○ E subarachnoid haemorrhage and xanthochromia after centrifugation

4. Tuberose sclerosis

- ○ A is an autosomal recessive condition
- ○ B is associated with renal angiomyolipomas in approximately 80% of people
- ○ C is excluded if the brain magnetic resonance imaging is normal
- ○ D is associated with retinal hamartomas
- ○ E is associated with autism

5. In acute disseminated encephalomyelitis

○ A unilateral optic neuritis is seen more commonly than in multiple sclerosis

○ B periventricular white matter lesions occur less commonly than in multiple sclerosis on magnetic resonance imaging

○ C a relapsing course is more common than in multiple sclerosis

○ D the EEG demonstrates excessive slow wave activity

○ E headache, fever and meningism are less common than in multiple sclerosis

6. Children with Rett syndrome

○ A have normal prenatal and perinatal development

○ B have a small head circumference at birth

○ C are usually female

○ D often fail to thrive

○ E show a mutation in *MECP-2*

7. The following neuromuscular disorders are correctly paired with their mode of inheritance

○ A myotonia congenita is autosomal dominant

○ B congenital muscular dystrophy is autosomal recessive

○ C facioscapulohumeral dystrophy is autosomal recessive

○ D Duchenne muscular dystrophy is X-linked dominant

○ E familial hyperkalaemic periodic paralysis is autosomal recessive

8. The following conditions are considered to be ion channelopathies

○ A episodic ataxia type 1

○ B autosomal dominant nocturnal frontal lobe epilepsy

○ C Lamberts–Eaton myasthenia

○ D hyperekplexia

○ E generalised epilepsy with febrile seizures (GEFS+)

9. Neonatal and childhood stroke

○ A ischaemic stroke results in a motor deficit in 75% of cases

○ B is as common as brain tumour

○ C is commonly treated by thrombolysis

○ D has a recurrence risk > 10%

○ E risk is increased in children with sickle cell anaemia

10. Febrile seizures

○ A the recurrence rate is greater than 50%

○ B have increased risk of recurrence if there is a family history of febrile convulsions

○   C   are associated with mesial temporal sclerosis
○   D   occur more often in children with neurodevelopmental abnormalities
○   E   should be investigated with EEG

11. Peripheral neuropathy is associated with

○   A   abetalipoproteinaemia
○   B   metachromatic leukodystrophy
○   C   amyloidosis
○   D   porphyria
○   E   ataxia telangiectasia

12. The following side effects of anti-epileptic drugs are well recognised

○   A   carbamazepine and hyponatraemia
○   B   valproate and weight loss
○   C   phenytoin and ataxia
○   D   lamotrigine and insomnia
○   E   topiramate and psychomotor slowing

13. In Sturge–Weber syndrome

○   A   there is a naevus in the distribution of the facial nerve
○   B   angiomas of the cortex occur in the occipital region
○   C   clinical seizures are focal and contralateral to the side of cerebral lesion
○   D   there is an association with hypocalcaemia
○   E   glaucoma is common

Best of Five Questions

14. An 8-year-old boy is found at night making salivatory and gurgling noises. He is unable to speak but seems conscious. His face is twitching on the left side. Which investigation is MOST likely to confirm the diagnosis?

- ○ A Brain CT with contrast
- ○ B Brain MRI
- ○ C EEG
- ○ D Thrombophilia screen
- ○ E Lumbar puncture

15. A newborn presents with a weak suck and weak cry. There is a fluctuating ptosis and hypotonia. The baby has attacks of apnoea. The mother has no medical history of note. The tests for anti-acetylcholine receptor antibodies are negative and there is a decremental response on repetitive nerve stimulation electromyography. The MOST likely diagnosis is?

- ○ A Transient neonatal myasthenia
- ○ B Autoimmune myasthenia
- ○ C Congenital myasthenia
- ○ D Möbius syndrome
- ○ E Spinal muscular atrophy type 1

16. An overweight 14-year-old girl has complained of headache on awakening for several weeks. She has papilloedema. Her blood pressure is normal. Brain MRI is normal. Which investigation is MOST likely to confirm the diagnosis?

- ○ A Sleep EEG
- ○ B CT brain with contrast
- ○ C Magnetic resonance spectroscopy
- ○ D Lumbar puncture with manometry
- ○ E Visual evoked responses and electroretinogram

17. The following signs are seen in a child with an ischaemic stroke: contralateral hemiparesis with face and arm more affected than the legs; horizontal gaze palsy and hemisensory deficits; language and cognitive deficits including aphasia and apraxia; homonymous hemianopia. Which artery is the MOST likely to be involved?

- ○ A Common carotid
- ○ B Middle cerebral
- ○ C Anterior cerebral
- ○ D Posterior cerebral
- ○ E Posterior cerebellar

18. A child presents with a facial palsy several weeks after a flu-like illness she had in the school holidays. She also has musculoskeletal pains and headache on direct questioning. On examination there is also splenomegaly and generalized lymphadenopathy. Which of the following investigations will be the MOST useful to aid diagnosis?

○ A *Borrelia* antibody serology
○ B Magnetic resonance imaging scan
○ C Anti-basal ganglia antibodies
○ D Stool culture for viruses
○ E Serum treponemal serologic tests

19. A 3-year-old boy presents with frequent falling. There is evidence of delay in motor milestones. He walked at 22 months. On examination he has a shuffling gait and foot drop. He has difficulty climbing stairs. Serum enzymes are normal. Nerve conduction studies are normal. CSF exam is normal. EMG reveals denervation and paucity of movement. The MOST likely diagnosis is which of the following?

○ A Type 2 spinal muscular atrophy
○ B Parkinson's disease
○ C Werdnig–Hoffman disease
○ D Emery–Dreifuss muscular dystrophy
○ E Kugelberg–Welander disease

20. An infant presents at age 4 months with hypotonia, weakness and constipation. On examination the pupillary responses are poorly reactive. Investigation reveals incremental response on rapid (20–50 Hz) repetitive nerve stimulation and abundant small motor unit potentials on electromyography. Tensilon test is negative. What is the MOST likely diagnosis?

○ A Spinal muscular atrophy
○ B Congenital myotonic dystrophy .
○ C Infantile botulism
○ D Congenital myopathy .
○ E Myasthenia gravis

21. **A 10-year-old girl presents with headache. It is unilateral, pulsating and rates 6/10 on the pain scale. The headache is worse on physical exercise and helped by sleep. Sometimes she sees photopsias. There is often nausea. What is the MOST likely diagnosis?**

- ○ A Cluster headache
- ○ B Tension headache
- ○ C Hydrocephalus
- ○ D Chronic paroxysmal hemicrania
- ○ E Classical migraine

22. **A child presents in a coma. There is central hyperventilation. Pupils are mid-position and irregular 3–5 mm and fixed. The vestibulo-ocular reflex is intact. He shows bilateral decerebrate posturing to noxious stimuli. What is MOST likely to be the position/location of the transtentorial herniation?**

- ○ A Reticular formation
- ○ B Diencephalon
- ○ C Mid-brain–upper pons
- ○ D Low pons–upper medulla
- ○ E Medulla

Extended Matching Questions

23. Theme: Anti-epileptic medication

A   Gabapentin
B   Sodium valproate
C   Phenytoin
D   Clonazepam
E   Carbamazepine
F   Lamotrigine
G   Levetiracetam
H   Phenobarbitone
I   Vigabatrin
J   Lorazepam

Select the most appropriate anti-epileptic medication for each of the following children. Each option may be used once, more than once, or not at all.

○   1. A 15-year-old boy seen in clinic who has had three witnessed generalised tonic–clonic seizures in the last 3 months.

○   2. A 4-year-old girl seen in clinic who has had several complex partial seizures.

○   3. A 6-month-old with infantile spasms and a chaotic hypsarrhythmic electroencephalogram. Woods light examination reveals several hypopigmented patches

24. Theme: EEG patterns in epilepsy syndromes

A   Hypsarrhythmia -
B   4–5 Hz poly-spike and wave discharges
C   Diffuse slow and spike wave discharges
D   Burst suppression pattern
E   Trace pointu alternans
F   Occipital spikes
G   Centrotemporal spikes
H   No abnormalities
I   Electrical status epilepticus in sleep
J   Unilateral temporal spikes

For the following epilepsy syndromes choose the most likely EEG pattern from those listed above. Each option may be used once, more than once, or not at all.

○   1. Juvenile absence epilepsy.
○   2. Lennox–Gastaut syndrome.
○   3. Landau–Kleffner syndrome.

25. Theme: Neurodegenerative disorders

A   Segawa disease
B   Hallervorden–Spatz syndrome
C   Huntington's chorea
D   Rasmussen's encephalitis
E   Sydenham's chorea
F   Ataxia telangiectasia
G   Wilson's disease
H   Subacute sclerosing panencephalitis
I   Lesch–Nyhan syndrome
J   Batten's disease

Match each of the following clinical scenarios with the most likely diagnosis. Each option may be used once, more than once, or not at all.

○   1. A child presents with a difficult to control focal seizure. On examination there is a hemianopia and hemiplegia. An EEG reveals diffuse paroxysmal activity with slow background and a brain MRI shows abnormalities in one hemisphere.

○   2. A 6-year-old boy presents following a period of normal development with rapid degeneration. Rigidity occurs in his lower limbs with equinovarus deformity in his feet. Choreoathetosis occurs in the muscles of the face, tongue and palate. Copper studies are normal. Ophthalmology is unremarkable.

○   3. A 6-year-old presents with intermittent toe walking and disturbed gait. There is diurnal variation in symptoms with improvement on awakening.

answers

1. Neurofibromatosis type 1

Answers: B D

Neurofibromatosis type 1 (NF 1) is an autosomal dominant condition with an incidence of 1 in 2500 to 1 in 3000. About half the cases are the first in the family. For diagnosis, two or more of the following are required:

- Six or more café-au-lait macules (> 0.5 cm in children and 1.5 cm in adults)
- Two or more cutaneous/subcutaneous neurofibromas, or one plexiform neurofibroma
- Axillary or groin freckling
- Optic pathway glioma
- Two or more Lisch nodules
- Bony dysplasia
- First degree relative with NF 1

Brain MRI is currently not recommended as a routine diagnostic test as the diagnosis is made by clinical assessment. MRI is currently not used for screening for optic glioma in the absence of progressive visual disturbance. Unidentified bright objects (UBOs) can be seen on MRI in children with NF 1, especially in children aged 8–16 years. These can help to confirm diagnosis in some cases. Plexiform neurofibromas undergo malignant change most commonly in the second and third decade in about 10% of cases. Optic gliomas are pilocytic astrocytomas that occur predominately in children under 7 years and are often indolent. Manifestations include optic atrophy, abnormal colour vision, squint, proptosis and hypothalamic disturbance.

2. Friedreich's ataxia

Answers: A B D

Friedreich's ataxia is the most common hereditary ataxia. The triplet repeat GAA is located in the first intron of the frataxin gene on chromosome 9q13. The frataxin protein is a mitochondrial protein that plays a part in iron homeostasis. Onset usually occurs around puberty with clumsiness of gait. Clinical features are: autosomal recessive onset prior to age 25 years, progressive limb and gait ataxia, absent tendon reflexes in the lower limbs, and evidence of axonal and sensory neuropathy on electrophysiological investigation. The motor nerve conduction velocities are usually normal. There is progression to dysarthria, areflexia, and loss of proprioception of distal joints, extensor plantars, and pyramidal weakness of the legs.

answers

3. Cerebrospinal fluid findings

Answers: A D E

CSF is produced mainly by the choroid plexus. It should have a clear and colourless appearance. Normal values in a child are as follows: protein 5–40 mg/dL; glucose 40–80 mg/dL with a CSF to blood ratio of 0.6; cell count < 5 × 10^9/mL. In tuberculous meningitis the glucose concentration will be decreased, with a high protein and increased cell count. In Guillain Barré, the protein can be normal or raised. Values peak between days 4 and 18. There are often oligoclonal bands that indicate local synthesis of immunoglobulin within the central nervous system. Oligoclonal bands can occur in multiple sclerosis, in sub-acute sclerosing panencephalitis and in Lyme disease. Xanthochromia occurs with cell counts above 500/mm³. This is a red–orange colouration of the CSF that occurs after breakdown of red blood cells. Oxyhaemoglobin is released and can be detected 2–4 hours after a subarachnoid bleed. It remains for 7–10 days. Xanthochromic CSF also occurs in hyperbilirubinaemia, hyperproteinaemia, hypercarotenaemia and with some drugs.

4. Tuberose sclerosis

Answers: B D E

Tuberose sclerosis is a common multisystem disorder affecting 1 in 5000 to 1 in 10, 000 newborns. Hamartomas or tumours most commonly affect brain, kidneys and skin. It is a dominantly inherited condition but 60–70% of cases are sporadic and represent new mutations. Two genes have been implicated, *TSC1* on chromosome 9 and *TSC2* on chromosome 16. Renal angiomyolipomas are benign hamartomas containing smooth muscle cells, blood vessels, and fat. They are often asymptomatic in children. By adulthood, complications can include renal failure, haemorrhage and mechanical obstruction. Normal imaging does not exclude the diagnosis and MRI is preferable to CT, although CT can be helpful to detect calcification. The predominant neurological manifestations include seizures, learning difficulties and behavioural problems.

5. Acute disseminated encephalomyelitis

Answer: D

Acute disseminated encephalomyelitis (ADEM) is the term given to a process in which there is disseminated inflammation at multiple sites within the central nervous system thought to occur at one point in time. Infections are often associated, especially those of the upper respiratory tract. Relapses can occur, and these are thought to represent part of the same acute immune process; the term multiphasic acute disseminated encephalomyelitis is used (MDEM). If, however, there appears to be a chronic immune process with relapses occurring in different sites at different times, a diagnosis of multiple sclerosis (MS) is made. There are many pathological and clinical similarities between ADEM and MS. In children, ADEM is diagnosed more frequently than MS. Some features help point towards ADEM as a diagnosis. Unilateral optic neuritis occurs less frequently in ADEM than in MS, for example. MRI can be useful. In ADEM there is relative sparing of periventricular white matter and follow up scans can show partial or complete resolution in contrast to MS where there may be new lesions. The EEG is frequently abnormal in both groups with slow-wave abnormalities being a non-specific sign of the encephalopathic process. The correct diagnosis is important as the risk of relapse and prognosis is very different between ADEM and MS and the best way to differentiate the conditions is the subject of ongoing research.

6. Rett syndrome

Answers: A C D E

Since the onset of genetic screening for the *MECP-2* gene on chromosome Xq28 the phenotype for Rett syndrome has been noted to be broad and non-specific. The inheritance is presumed to be X-linked dominant with early male lethality. Supportive criteria for diagnosis include loss of acquired skills, acquired microcephaly, developmental delay, and autistic features with stereotypic hand movements. The head growth usually slows between 2–4 months of age but is often unrecognised. Failure to thrive is common in children with Rett syndrome. Dysfunctional swallowing may necessitate gastrostomy tube placement. Fluid intake needs to be increased to compensate for drooling and hyperventilation.

7. Inheritance of neuromuscular disorders

Answers: A B

Facioscapulohumeral dystrophy (FSH) is autosomal dominant and shows marked clinical variation. It must be carefully differentiated from some of the forms of congenital myopathy. Duchenne muscular dystrophy is the most common and one of most severe forms of muscular dystrophy and is an X-linked recessive condition due to a mutation on chromosome Xp21. The mutation results in a lack of dystrophin protein. About a third of cases arise as new mutations. Familial periodic paralysis is autosomal dominant.

8. Ion channelopathies

Answers: All true

Neurons, nerves and muscles communicate through electrical impulses mediated by rapid transit of ions through channels. Many disorders have their basis in dysfunction of ion channels. Channelopathies are sub-divided according to the ion channel involved in the molecular defect. The symptoms are often paroxysmal but are often associated with progressive dysfunction and disability. Sodium channelopathies include the autosomal dominant

answers

conditions hyperkalaemic periodic paralysis and paramyotonia congenita. Potassium channelopathies include Andersen syndrome (dysmorphism, ventricular arrhythmia and periodic paralysis). Chloride and calcium channel disorders are also well described.

9. Neonatal and childhood stroke

Answers: A B D E

Childhood stroke is as common as brain tumour, occurring in 2.5 to 13 per 100, 000 children and in 40 per 100, 000 neonates. Around half the children presenting with ischaemic arterial stroke will have sickle cell anaemia or congenital cardiac disease. Other predisposing conditions include immunodeficiency, homocystinuria and bacterial meningitis. In the neonate the pathology usually suggests an embolic aetiology. Venous sinus thrombosis is particularly common in the neonate although it can occur at all ages. Haemorrhagic stroke may be caused by coagulopathies or structural lesions such as arteriovenous malformation. There has been an argument to give thrombolysis for ischaemic stroke within the first 3 hours. Very few children will present within this recommended time to a stroke centre for accurate assessment and management. Around 75% of children with ischaemic stroke have a residual motor deficit. They may also present with cognitive and behavioural difficulties. Modifiable risk factors need to be identified to prevent recurrence.

10. Febrile seizures

Answers: B C D

Febrile seizures are one of the commonest neurological disorders of childhood. The diagnosis is clinical and an EEG is not indicated. The outcome is usually good. The recurrence risk for febrile convulsions is increased by between 20–40% in younger ages and if there is a family history of febrile convulsions. The risk of epilepsy following febrile seizures is multiplied by a factor of four when compared to the population. Risk factors for epilepsy include positive family history, and prolonged or atypical febrile seizures. Remember, in children with epilepsy fever may lower the seizure threshold.

11. Neuropathy

Answer: All true

Hereditary neuropathies constitute a complex heterogeneous group of disorders. They frequently have insidious onset and slow indolent progression. There are several main groups – a few examples are: hereditary motor and sensory neuropathies, such as Charcot–Marie–Tooth; predominantly sensory neuropathies (types I to IV); ataxic neuropathies such as giant axonal neuropathy; metabolic disorders; and degenerative disorders with peripheral nerve involvement. The question includes examples of conditions associated with neuropathy

12. Side effects of anti-epileptic drugs

Answers: A C D E

There are many side effects listed for each of the anti-epileptic drugs but these are some of the more commonly reported ones. Valproate is associated with weight gain, hepatic enzyme elevation, alopecia and tremor; it can also cause thrombocytopenia and hyperammonaemia. Carbamazepine can cause the syndrome of inappropriate anti-diuretic hormone (SIADH) and therefore low sodium; other side effects are diplopia, vertigo, sedation, headache and stomatitis. Phenytoin can cause drowsiness, ataxia, diplopia, hypotension, hirsutism and gingival hyperplasia to list just a few. Lamotrigine may cause rashes, dizziness, and ataxia, as well as headache, vomiting and insomnia. Speech disorders, renal stones and sedation are side effects of topiramate, as well as psychomotor slowing.

13. In Sturge–Weber syndrome

Answers: B C E

Sturge–Weber is a syndrome that includes facial nacvus in the trigeminal distribution, hemiparesis, unilateral seizures and in more than half of cases learning difficulties. Calcium deposition occurs adjacent to abnormal vessels often termed tramline calcification on X-ray.

14. C: Electroencephalogram (EEG)

This is the typical presentation of a child with rolandic epilepsy, also termed benign childhood epilepsy with centrotemporal spikes. It is also common to have brief daytime hemi-facial twitching with increased salivation. This is a common condition accounting for about 15% of children with afebrile seizures. It can be recognised on clinical grounds and has a distinctive EEG.

15. C: Congenital myasthenia

The clues to the diagnosis of myasthenia are the fluctuation of weakness and the decremental response with repetitive nerve stimulation EMG. There are three main groups of myasthenic syndromes: the autoimmune form (often known as juvenile myasthenia), congenital myasthenia gravis (sometimes called genetic), and transient neonatal myasthenia. The latter is due to transplacental passage of antibody to the acetylcholine receptor in mothers with myasthenia gravis. Clearance of antibody can take 5 months after birth. Congenital myasthenic syndromes are a heterogeneous group and the defect can be pre-synaptic, synaptic and post-synaptic. It is important to remember these in the differential diagnosis of apnoea in the newborn. Spinal muscular atrophy type 1 involves degeneration of motor neurons. There is symmetrical weakness caused by denervation, with associated muscle atrophy. The neonate often will present with hypotonia, but the face is usually strong with full movement. There is no loss of sensation. The EMG demonstrates a neuropathic reduced recruitment of voluntary muscle unit potentials. Molecular analysis is now used to make the diagnosis and over 95% of cases have deletions in the survival motor neuron (*SMN*) gene. Möbius syndrome is characterized by bilateral facial weakness. There is often paralysis of the abducens nerve associated with it.

16. D: Lumbar puncture with manometry

Benign intracranial hypertension is a headache syndrome showing raised cerebrospinal fluid pressure in absence of mass lesion or dilated ventricles. There are usually normal findings on examination except for papilloedema and occasional VIth nerve palsy. The condition requires close monitoring of visual acuity as optic nerve damage can occur as a result of chronically raised pressure. Treatment can involve repeat lumbar punctures to remove cerebrospinal fluid, acetazolamide and analgesics.

17. B: Middle cerebral

Common carotid occlusion may be asymptomatic. The anterior cerebral artery occlusions present with contralateral hemiparesis involving the leg to a greater extent than the arm and face. There can be a contralateral grasp reflex and gait disorders. Urinary incontinence is a feature. Posterior cerebral artery occlusions involve contralateral homonymous hemianopia. There may be memory loss and dyslexia.

18. A: *Borrelia* antibody serology

This clinical presentation is consistent with the diagnosis of Lyme disease. This is a multisystem disorder caused by a tick-transmitted spirochete, *Borrelia burgdorferi*. Localized infection occurs following a tick bite, which is often forgotten about or not noticed. This is followed by disseminated infection for up to 9 months. Late or persistent infection can occur for months or years. Neurological manifestations include progressive encephalomyelitis, focal encephalitis, dementia, seizures and polyneuropathy.

19. E: Kugelberg–Welander disease

The usual onset of Kugelberg–Welander disease is after 2 years and children have often walked late. There is slow deterioration that results in scoliosis and wheelchair dependence. Type 2 spinal muscular atrophy, Werdnig–Hoffman disease, and Kugelberg–Welander disease are all forms of spinal muscular atrophy, each having degeneration in the anterior horn cell of the spinal cord, and in some cases the motor nuclei of the brainstem. Type 1 is the most severe form and can present with reduced fetal movements or neonatal hypotonia. Type 2 is intermediate severity but the children are usually unable to walk unaided. Muscle biopsy and molecular genetic studies for the *SMN* gene confirms the diagnosis. Parkinson's disease rarely presents in childhood.

20. C: Infantile botulism

The conditions listed above can all present with peripheral hypotonia. Infant botulism most commonly presents at 2–6 months with the symptoms described above. *Clostridium botulinum* is a Gram-positive spore-forming organism found in soil, agricultural products, and honey. Respiratory failure can occur. The toxin is released and binds irreversibly to pre-synaptic cholinergic nerve terminals and disrupts the exocytosis of acetylcholine. Positive stool culture or isolation of toxin is difficult because of constipation. Management is supportive. Pupillary responses should not be affected in the other conditions. A positive Tensilon test would be expected with myasthenia syndromes. The EMG in congenital myotonic dystrophy may demonstrate myotonic potentials firing at high rates that wax and wane in frequency and amplitude.

21. E: Classical migraine

Headache disorders are common in childhood. This is a description of classic migraine with aura of flashing lights. Cluster headaches are more common in males, most often occurring in those in their late 20s and rarely in children. Periodicity is the predominant feature with chronic episodes of headaches lasting for 2–3 months; there is usually no aura, and the pain is excruciating often in the trigeminal distribution and may be associated with lacrimation, sweating, ptosis and nasal congestion. Tension headaches are diffuse and bilateral often described as pressing or a being like a tight band; auras are rare. Chronic paroxysmal hemicrania is similar to cluster headache but the pain is usually in or around the orbit; headaches last for a short time (5 minutes) but occur many times a day. Hydrocephalus can present as headache. This is usually worse in the morning. There may be associated gait abnormalities and cranial nerve signs notably VIth nerve palsy and diplopia. There is often loss of fine motor coordination. Papilloedema is frequently present.

22. C: Mid-brain–upper pons

There is a rostral–caudal progression of signs seen with both lateral and central transtentorial herniation, indicating worsening of the herniation. This begins with diencephalic involvement followed by mesencephalic, pontine, and finally medullary involvement. The signs described above are seen with involvement of the mid-brain and upper pons. With herniation at the level of the reticular formation there is altered consciousness. With involvement of the diencephalon there is drowsiness or agitation with Cheyne–Stokes respirations. Pupils are small but brisk. Eye movements can be roving, the vestibulo-ocular reflex is weak or brisk. There is loss of vertical movement.

answers

Decorticate posturing to stimuli occurs. Plantars are extensor. With involvement of the low pons–upper medulla the patient will be in a coma with tachypnoea. Small mid-position fixed pupils are present. Vestibulo-ocular reflex is absent. There is flaccid flexor response to noxious stimuli. With involvement of the medulla the patient will be in coma. Breathing will become apnoeic, then stop. Pupils are fixed and dilated. There is no vestibulo-ocular reflex. Limbs are flaccid with no deep tendon reflexes.

23. ANTI-EPILEPTIC MEDICATION

The identification of a seizure type and or an epilepsy syndrome provides information on prognosis and guides the choice of drug treatment when this is deemed appropriate. It is always important to consider the safety profile of the treatment and available formulation. Monotherapy at the lowest dosage to achieve control is the ideal with any drug treatment.

1.   B – Sodium valproate

For idiopathic generalised epilepsies sodium valproate is usually first-line choice of medication. The exception is for teenaged girls because it is necessary to consider the risk of polycystic ovaries as well as teratogenicity. Lamotrigine would be preferred in this group.

2.   E – Carbamazepine

Carbamazepine is first-line therapy for partial seizure disorders.

3.   I – Vigabatrin

West syndrome is characterized by infantile spasms, hypsarrhythmia and developmental delay. The first-line medications for this group are prednisolone, adrenocorticotrophic hormone, or vigabatrin. With an underlying diagnosis of tuberose sclerosis vigabatrin is preferred.

24. EEG PATTERNS IN EPILEPSY SYNDROMES

1.   B – 4–5 Hz poly-spike and wave discharges

Juvenile absence epilepsy begins in the early part of the second decade. Absences are less frequent but may be longer than in childhood absence epilepsy. Generalized tonic–clonic seizures (GTC) often occur. The frequency of the spike wave discharges is often faster than the 3 Hz seen in childhood absence epilepsy.

2.   C – Diffuse slow and spike wave discharges

Lennox–Gastaut is the best-known example of symptomatic generalized epilepsy. Multiple aetiologies have been identified including tuberose sclerosis, cerebral dysgenesis and Batten's disease. Seizure types include GTC, absences, drop attacks, and myoclonic jerks. Characteristic EEG is general irregular 1.5–2.5 Hz sharp and slow-wave activity with slow background. During sleep, bursts of sharp discharges around 10 Hz can occur.

3.   I – Electrical status epilepticus in sleep

Landau–Kleffner is an acquired epileptic aphasia in which regression of language skills occurs. The EEG abnormalities can show multifocal spike or spike and wave in the temporoparietal region whilst awake, and frequent generalized spike wave discharges (ESES, electrical status epilepticus) in sleep.

25. NEURODEGENERATIVE DISORDERS

1. D – Rasmussen's encephalitis

Rasmussen's encephalitis typically presents with focal seizures which can be frequent or even continuous. Rasmussen described a syndrome of seizures, spastic paralysis and learning difficulties associated with chronic encephalitis. The brain imaging can be normal early in the disease. Later in the course, cerebral swelling can be seen with high intensity lesions in the basal ganglia and periventricular white matter on T2-weighted imaging. The diagnosis would need to be confirmed on brain biopsy in a clinically suspected case.

2. B – Hallervorden–Spatz syndrome

Hallervorden–Spatz is a rare degenerative disorder inherited as a recessive trait. There is usually progressive dystonia, rigidity and choreoathetosis. Death usually occurs by early adulthood. Imaging shows lesions of the globus pallidus. Neuropathology reveals excess accumulation of iron-containing pigments in the globus pallidus and substantia nigra.

3. A – Segawa disease

Segawa disease is otherwise known as dopa-responsive dystonia due to the clinical response. It is more common in females and typically presents around the age of 6 years with dystonic posturing of the lower limb. It improves with a small dose of levodopa.

Ophthalmology

Mike Champion

1. **The following is true of retinitis pigmentosa**
   - ○ A the disease process predominantly affects the cones
   - ○ B it is a recognised feature of Laurence–Moon–Biedl syndrome
   - ○ C night blindness is a presenting feature
   - ○ D central scotoma is the characteristic resultant visual field defect
   - ○ E disease progression is significantly retarded by vitamin C supplementation

2. **The following present with a painful red eye**
   - ○ A juvenile rheumatoid arthritis
   - ○ B *Toxocara canis* infection
   - ○ C glaucoma
   - ○ D herpes simplex
   - ○ E toxoplasmosis

3. **The features of acquired Horner syndrome in a 3-year-old child following cardiac surgery include**
   - ○ A mydriasis
   - ○ B ptosis
   - ○ C ipsilateral anhydrosis
   - ○ D normal pupillary reflexes
   - ○ E heterochromia iridis

4. **Glaucoma is a recognised complication of the following**
   - ○ A Wilson disease
   - ○ B Horner syndrome
   - ○ C retinopathy of prematurity
   - ○ D Marfan syndrome
   - ○ E neurofibromatosis type 1

5. The following are causes of congenital cataracts

- A maternal diabetes
- B galactosaemia
- C varicella zoster
- D hypothyroidism
- E maternal steroids

6. The following is true of retinoblastoma

- A leukocoria is the most common presenting sign
- B the affected eye is usually painful
- C most cases result from a sporadic mutation in the retinoblastoma gene
- D the risk of recurrence in unilateral disease in the unaffected eye is 10%
- E patients are at risk of developing secondary malignant tumours at distant sites in later life

7. Blue sclerae are a recognised feature of the following

- A osteogenesis imperfecta
- B trisomy 21
- C Ehlers–Danlos syndrome
- D β-thalassaemia
- E ataxia telangiectasia

8. The following are inherited in an autosomal recessive fashion

- A Leber's hereditary optic neuropathy
- B keratoconus
- C Waardenburg syndrome
- D Leber's amaurosis
- E Joubert syndrome

9. In congenital rubella syndrome

- A infection in the first trimester is associated with the greatest likelihood of an affected fetus
- B pregnant seronegative women should be immediately immunized
- C cataract is the commonest ocular feature
- D the presence of rubella IgG antibodies in the infant confirms the diagnosis
- E the electroretinogram is usually normal

10. In orbital cellulitis

- A blood cultures are often negative
- B *Staphylococcus aureus* is the most common cause in infancy
- C incidence is greatest in children over 5 years
- D investigation includes sinus X-ray
- E intravenous antibiotics alone are sufficient to clear the majority of cases

11. In chlamydial conjunctivitis

○ A oral erythromycin is the treatment of choice
○ B cytoplasmic inclusion bodies are characteristic
○ C it usually presents within 48 hours of birth
○ D asymptomatic parents require treatment
○ E concurrent pneumonitis is common

12. Ptosis is a feature of

○ A Möbius syndrome
○ B Kearns–Sayre syndrome
○ C abducens palsy
○ D collodion baby
○ E Marcus–Gunn jaw winking syndrome

13. Vernal conjunctivitis

○ A is commoner in girls
○ B is associated with atopy
○ C is seasonal
○ D requires long-term corticosteroid use
○ E has photophobia as a common feature

14. Risk factors for retinopathy of prematurity include

○ A birth weight less than 1000 g
○ B female
○ C blood transfusions
○ D pre-term gestation
○ E intracranial haemorrhage

15. Leukocoria is a recognised feature of

○ A cataract
○ B toxocariasis
○ C retinoblastoma
○ D Hurler syndrome
○ E persistent hyperplastic primary vitreous

Best of Five Questions

16. **What is the MOST likely visual field defect in a child diagnosed with craniopharyngioma?**

    ○ A Blindness in one eye
    ○ B Homonymous hemianopia
    ○ C Bitemporal hemianopia
    ○ D Peripheral field defect
    ○ E Central scotoma

17. **A 2-day-old neonate develops a copious purulent discharge with associated lid swelling. What is the MOST likely causative organism?**

    ○ A *Chlamydia*
    ○ B *Neisseria gonorrhoeae*
    ○ C *Haemophilus influenzae*
    ○ D *Staphylococcus aureus*
    ○ E Herpes simplex

18. **Examination of the pupillary light reflex in the left eye of a 7-year-old girl reveals an absent direct reflex and normal consensual reflex. These findings are MOST consistent with which one of the following?**

    ○ A Left oculomotor nerve palsy
    ○ B Right oculomotor nerve palsy
    ○ C Left Horner syndrome
    ○ D Left optic nerve lesion
    ○ E Right optic nerve lesion

19. **What is the treatment of choice for *Toxocara canis* infection in a 3-year-old boy presenting with leukocoria. Fundoscopy reveals a large lesion close to the macula with marked inflammation.**

    ○ A Cryotherapy
    ○ B Corticosteroids
    ○ C Laser therapy
    ○ D Observation
    ○ E Antihelminthic drugs

questions

20. **Viral conjunctivitis is MOST commonly caused by which of the following?**

○ A Adenovirus
○ B Herpes simplex
○ C Paramyxovirus
○ D Corona virus
○ E Coxsackie virus

21. **A 5-year-old child presents with acute onset ophthalmoplegia of the right eye with associated proptosis and ptosis following a heavy head cold. The MOST likely diagnosis is which of the following?**

○ A Orbital cellulitis
○ B Mastoiditis
○ C Cavernous sinus thrombosis
○ D Frontal sinusitis
○ E Cerebral abscess

22. **The MOST appropriate test for assessing acuity in a 3-year-old child is which of the following?**

○ A Sheridan Gardner test
○ B Standard Snellen chart
○ C Catford drum
○ D Preferential looking test
○ E Graded rolling ball test

Extended Matching Questions

23. Theme: Eye movements

A   Abduction of the right eye
B   Adduction of the right eye
C   Abduction of the right eye on upgaze
D   Adduction of the right eye on upgaze
E   Abduction of the right eye on downgaze
F   Adduction of the right eye on downgaze
G   Upgaze
H   Downgaze
I   All directions

For the three causes of disconjugate eye movements described below, select the position of the eye where diplopia is maximal from those listed above. Each option may be used once, more than once, or not at all.

○ 1. Right-sided Brown's syndrome.
○ 2. Right-sided abducens nerve palsy.
○ 3. Right-sided trochlear nerve palsy.

24. Theme: Masses around the eye

A   Rhabdomyoma
B   Hordeolum
C   Neuroblastoma
D   Cyst of Moll
E   Meibomian cyst
F   Dermoid
G   Obstructed tear duct
H   Capillary haemangioma
I   Cavernous sinus thrombosis

Select the best option from the list above to match the following descriptions of masses around the eye. Each option may be used once, more than once, or not at all.

○ 1. A painless hard nodule in an 8-year-old boy near the upper-lid margin that has been present for some weeks, but has recently become red and inflamed.
○ 2. A tender red superficial swelling on the outer eyelid margin in a 3-year-old girl.
○ 3. A 4-day-old boy presents with a bluish mass inferior to the medial canthus.

25. Theme: Drug adverse effects

A   Phenytoin
B   Amiodarone
C   Paracetamol
D   Ibuprofen
E   Ethambutol
F   Rifampicin
G   Vigabatrin
H   Corticosteroids
I   Insulin

Match the following adverse effects to the drugs listed above. Each option may be used once, more than once, or not at all.

○ 1. Visual field defect.
○ 2. Colour blindness.
○ 3. Corneal deposits.

answers

1. Retinitis pigmentosa

Answers: B C

Retinitis pigmentosa is a progressive disorder predominantly affecting rod cells, and therefore poor night vision with abnormal dark adaptation is a common presenting symptom. Peripheral vision is affected first, where the rods are concentrated, resulting in sparing of the central vision and the development of tunnel vision. Around 50% of cases are sporadic, 20% are recessive, 20% are dominant and 10% are X-linked. Associations include abetalipoproteinaemia, Refsum syndrome, Laurence–Moon–Biedl syndrome, mitochondrial disorders, Friedreich's ataxia, neuronal ceroid lipofuscinosis, Usher syndrome, and Chediak–Higashi disease. The retinitis pigmentosa of abetalipoproteinaemia may respond to vitamin E supplementation.

2. Painful red eye

Answers: A C D

The uveal tract consists of the iris, ciliary body, and choroid. Anterior uveitis (anterior chamber and iris) and pan-uveitis are painful, whereas posterior uveitis (choroid and retina) is painless, and therefore disease progression may be more marked prior to diagnosis in young children. Causes of posterior uveitis include infection by *Toxocara* and *Toxoplasma*.

3. Horner syndrome following cardiac surgery

Answers: B C D

Horner syndrome results from a lack of sympathetic innervation of the pupil. The pupil is constricted (miosis) with ipsilateral ptosis. Heterochromia is a feature of congenital Horner syndrome or early surgery involving the eye in the first year. Pupillary reflexes are normal.

4. Glaucoma

Answers: C D E

Glaucoma (raised intra-ocular pressure) results in expansion of the eye size in infants under 3 years of age, and damage of the optic nerve head. Congenital glaucoma results from abnormal drainage of the anterior chamber due to abnormal angle structures. Secondary causes include eye diseases that affect the anatomy making outflow obstruction more likely, and these include aniridia, Sturge–Weber syndrome, Lowe syndrome, neurofibromatosis type 1, Marfan syndrome, retinopathy of prematurity, and rubella syndrome.

5. Congenital cataracts

Answers: All true

50% of congenital cataracts are idiopathic. The most common identifiable cause of congenital cataract is autosomal dominant inherited cataract, and therefore the parental history and examination need to be thorough. Other causes include maternal disease such as diabetes, and the maternal ingestion of exogenous steroids. Intra-uterine infections (3%) and systemic disease (5%) account for only a small number of cases.

6. Retinoblastoma

Answers: A C E

Retinoblastoma arises from the retina usually presenting with leukocoria (white pupil) or squint. Usually the disease is painless, unless tumour necrosis results in inflammation. Calcification is common and can be detected by CT scan of the orbits. The retinoblastoma gene is located on chromosome 13 and is a growth suppressor gene. Disease results from a double hit. In hereditary cases, one affected gene is inherited and the second undergoes mutation after conception. Sporadic cases result from spontaneous mutation of both genes. Cure rates are 90% in uni-ocular disease. Large tumours require enucleation. Smaller tumours can be treated with radiotherapy or chemotherapy The risk of recurrence in the unaffected eye is 20%, and falls markedly after 2 years. Patients are at risk of developing late secondary tumours, even at distant sites.

7. Blue sclerae

Answers: A C

Blue sclerae are not the soul preserve of osteogenesis imperfecta, but are also seen in other conditions with connective tissue involvement. These include Ehlers–Danlos syndrome, hypophosphatasia, Marfan syndrome, Turner syndrome, and trisomy 18.

Blue sclerae are seen in the most severe osteogenesis imperfecta (types I and II) and are not a feature of the milder dominantly inherited forms. The bluish appearance results from thinning of the sclera, which allows the black choroid to be slightly visible. β-thalassaemia is associated with icteric sclerae secondary to haemolysis.

8. Autosomal recessive inheritance

Answers: D E

Leber's amaurosis is an autosomal recessive, childhood onset, retinal degeneration that results in blindness from birth or early childhood. Joubert syndrome is similarly inherited; this consists of retinal dystrophy, cerebellar vermis hypoplasia, nystagmus and episodic tachypnoea. Leber's hereditary optic neuropathy is a mitochondrial disorder resulting from a mtDNA point mutation. It is characterised by painless acute or subacute bilateral central

answers

vision loss occurring in the second to fourth decade. It is more common in males. Keratoconus is sporadic, or dominant in < 10% of cases. There is corneal thinning, which results in localised protrusion, producing irregular astigmatism and myopia. Waardenburg syndrome is an autosomal dominant condition with sensorineural hearing loss, facial dysmorphism, and abnormal pigmentation of eyes, hair, and skin.

9. Congenital rubella syndrome

Answers: A E

The risk of congenital rubella syndrome diminishes as the pregnancy progresses, and the full syndrome is rare if the infection occurs after the fourth month of the pregnancy. Seronegative pregnant women should be immunised post-partum. Pigmentary retinopathy is the most common ocular manifestation, however the electroretinogram is usually normal, indicating that the pigmentary mottling does not affect the retinal pigmentary epithelium. Diagnosis is confirmed on isolation of the virus from nasopharyngeal aspirates, from urine, or cerebrospinal fluid. IgG antibodies may be maternal in origin. The presence of both IgG and IgM antibodies suggests recent infection. Cataract occurs in 20–30% of patients.

10. Orbital cellulitis

Answers: A C D E

Orbital cellulitis occurs most commonly in children aged over 5 years, compared to pre-septal cellulitis (cellulitis involving the external soft tissues and eyelid) which is more common in younger infants (mean age 8 months). 90% of cases are secondary to sinusitis and therefore sinus X-rays are essential. Some advocate computerised tomographic imaging, which shows sub-periosteal and orbital abscesses that are not apparent on plain films. *Haemophilus* is the commonest organism in infants, and high-dose intravenous cephalosporin is the treatment of choice, curing over 60% of cases. Fungal orbital cellulitis is associated with immunodeficiency and diabetes.

11. Chlamydial conjunctivitis

Answers: A B D

Chlamydial conjunctivitis typically presents after 48 hours, unlike gonococcal conjunctivitis, and may present as late as 14 days or more. Diagnosis is confirmed on Giemsa staining of conjunctival scrapings to reveal cytoplasmic inclusion bodies. Oral erythromycin is the treatment of choice having the advantage over topical treatment of clearing nasopharyngeal carriage, reducing the risk of recurrence. Parents – even if asymptomatic – require treatment. Pneumonitis occurs in approximately 10–20% of cases, and usually presents much later, between 3 and 11 weeks.

12. Ptosis

Answers: A B E

Möbius syndrome results from a combination of facial nerve (VIIth) and abducens (VIth) nerve palsy and is often associated with an oculomotor (IIIrd) nerve palsy. An isolated VIth nerve palsy causes failure of abduction of the eye, but does not affect the lid. Kearns–Sayre is a mitochondrial disorder with progressive external ophthalmoplegia (reduction of gaze in all directions), ptosis, pigmentary retinopathy, and heart block. A collodion baby is covered with a tense cellophane-like membrane resulting in ectropion as the tissues around the eyes are held in traction. The ptosis of Marcus–Gunn jaw winking syndrome resolves on mouth opening and lateral movement of the jaw. It results from aberrant innervation of the levator muscle of the eyelid from the trigeminal (Vth) nerve.

13. Vernal conjunctivitis

Answers: B C E

Vernal conjunctivitis is a severe allergic condition presenting with intense itching, tearing, mucus production, and giant papillae on the upper tarsal conjunctiva. Secondary keratitis during exacerbations causes photophobia. The condition is seasonal, often starting in spring and is commoner in boys, usually starting in those under 10 years of age. 90% of cases have other allergic diseases in addition to an atopic family history. Treatment is based on mast cell stabilisers (cromoglycate drops) and topical antihistamines. Severe exacerbations may necessitate topical steroids but long-term use is to be avoided to prevent secondary glaucoma or cataracts.

14. Retinopathy of prematurity

Answers: A C D E

Risk factors for retinopathy of prematurity include low birth weight, hyperoxia, respiratory distress syndrome, intracranial haemorrhage, pre-term gestation, and blood transfusions. The incidence increases dramatically with birth weights of less than 1000 g. Adult haemoglobin dissociates oxygen more readily than fetal haemoglobin, therefore transfusions increase retinal oxygen dose. Gender is not a risk factor.

15. Leukocoria

Answers: A B C E

Leukocoria is defined as a white pupil and is indicative of an opacity at or behind the pupil (of the lens, vitreous or retina). The differential diagnosis includes cataract, retinoblastoma, toxocariasis, persistent hyperplastic primary vitreous, myelinated nerve fibres, and retinopathy or prematurity. Hurler syndrome and the mucopolysaccharidoses – with the exception of Hunter syndrome – are associated with corneal clouding.

16. C: Bitemporal hemianopia

Craniopharyngioma may be suprasellar, or supra- and intrasellar, and therefore as the tumour increases in size, pressure is applied to the optic chiasm. This is the site of decussation of the temporal field fibres and therefore vision in the temporal fields is lost bilaterally.

17. B: *Neisseria gonorrhoeae*

The very early onset makes *Neisseria gonorrhoeae* the most likely organism, usually presenting on day 2–4 of life. *Staphylococcus* and *Streptococcus* cause purulent neonatal conjunctivitis, but present later (day 4–7). *Chlamydia* produces a serous or purulent discharge (day 4–10). *Haemophilus* tends to be a serous discharge (onset 5–10 days) as does herpes simplex, but the onset is much later (6 days to 2 weeks).

18. D: Left optic nerve lesion

The findings are consistent with damage to the optic nerve in the affected eye. In IIIrd nerve palsy the pupil is fixed dilated and does not react to direct or consensual light. In Horner syndrome the pupils are small due to the interrupted sympathetic supply to the pupillary dilator muscle, but are able to constrict to light.

19. B: Corticosteroids

The siting of the lesion requires active management. Steroids are the preferred choice, either systemic or periocular. Small peripheral lesions may be observed. The use of antihelminthic drugs is controversial as death of the larva can exacerbate the inflammation, and steroids would still be prescribed. Laser therapy has been advocated but it has the same increased risk of inflammation following death of the larva.

20. A: Adenovirus

Viral conjunctivitis is usually caused by adenovirus and is very contagious. First one eye is involved, and this then spreads to the other. Signs and symptoms include tearing, redness, and the sensation of having a foreign body in the eye. If the cornea becomes involved, then photophobia can develop.

21. C: Cavernous sinus thrombosis

The main differential is between orbital cellulitis and cavernous sinus thrombosis. However, the latter is suggested by the acute onset of reduction in eye movements. The ophthalmoplegia is secondary to IIIrd, IVth and VIth nerve involvement, all of which pass through the cavernous sinus. Eye movements may be slightly reduced secondary to pain in orbital cellulitis. Treatment consists of intravenous antibiotics and/or drainage of sinuses if they are the source of infection. Frontal sinusitis presents with tenderness over the forehead and may be the source of the infection along with sphenoid and the ethmoid sinuses. Mastoiditis presents with swelling over the mastoid air cells behind the ear. A cerebral abscess is more likely to present with altered consciousness, vomiting and pyrexia.

22. A: Sheridan Gardner test

In the Sheridan Gardner test, the child has a key card with five letters. The examiner stands 6 m away and holds up letters of different size which the child has to match with those on the card. A standard Snellen chart can usually be used in children aged 7 years upwards. The other three tests are used for testing in pre-verbal children. The Catford drum (vertical stripes) relies on normal acuity to produce optokinetic nystagmus.

23. EYE MOVEMENTS

1. D – Adduction of the right eye on upgaze

Brown's syndrome results from a congenitally tight superior oblique muscle tendon complex. This means that the eye fails to elevate in adduction. Patients may develop a compensatory chin lift and may slightly turn their face away from the affected eye.

2. A – Abduction of the right eye

The abducens (VIth) nerve innervates the lateral rectus muscle which abducts the eye.

3. E – Abduction of the right eye on downgaze

The trochlear (IVth) nerve innervates the superior oblique muscle, which acts to depress and intort (twist nasally) the eye. Patients usually present with head tilt to the opposite side. This is common congenitally or from trauma.

24. MASSES AROUND THE EYE

1. E – Meibomian cyst

Meibomian glands are sebaceous glands with their opening at the lid margin. Their function is to reduce evaporation of tears by covering the tear film with sterol esters and waxes. Blockage of the gland results in swelling (chalazion). If it fails to resolve after several weeks, drainage may be necessary.

2. B – Hordeolum

Hordeolum (stye) is an abscess of an eyelash follicle which therefore appears as a tender swelling at the eyelid margin. A cyst of Moll lies on the anterior eyelid margin, but is painless and translucent.

3. G – Obstructed tear duct

Infants with nasolacrimal duct obstruction present with tearing and increased mucus accumulating at the inner canthus. Spontaneous resolution occurs in half of all cases by 6 months. An amniotocele may appear as a swelling in the medial canthal area as a result of fluid sequestered in the nasolacrimal sac. If not infected, local massage may affect a cure. Infection requires intravenous antibiotics and probing.

answers

25. DRUG ADVERSE EFFECTS

1. G – Vigabatrin

Vigabatrin may cause permanent visual field loss, and therefore an attempt should be made to assess baseline perimetry prior to – or soon after – starting treatment, and every 6 months thereafter.

2. E – Ethambutol

Ethambutol is used to treat tuberculosis. Retrobulbar neuritis is a dose-dependent side effect that presents with colour vision defects, central and paracentral scotoma, and reduced acuity. Recovery may take weeks to months after ethambutol is stopped.

3. B – Amiodarone

Amiodarone deposits are seen in both lens and cornea, and are related both to dose and duration of treatment. The deposits are reversible.

Respiratory medicine

Andrew Clark

Multiple Choice Questions

1. Erythema nodosum is a recognised feature of
- A sarcoidosis
- B cystic fibrosis
- C pneumococcal pneumonia
- D pulmonary tuberculosis
- E Kawasaki's disease

2. The oxyhaemoglobin dissociation curve is shifted to the right in the following situation(s)
- A increase in temperature
- B hypocarbia
- C alkalosis
- D increase in D-2,3–diphosphoglycerate
- E carbon monoxide poisoning

3. In transfer of gas across the alveolar capillary membrane
- A oxygen diffuses more rapidly than carbon dioxide
- B rate of gas transfer is proportional to solubility
- C rate of gas transfer is proportional to capillary area
- D gases with a higher molecular weight diffuse across more rapidly
- E type I pneumocytes comprise 95% of the alveolar surface

4. Digital clubbing is a characteristic feature of
- A cystic fibrosis
- B pulmonary sequestration
- C bronchopulmonary dysplasia
- D primary ciliary dysplasia
- E biliary cirrhosis

5. Nasal polyps are a recognised feature of

- ○ A Wegener's granulomatosis
- ○ B chronic rhinitis
- ○ C Aspirin sensitivity
- ○ D cystic fibrosis
- ○ E hypothyroidism

6. Percentage of predicted FEV$_1$

- ○ A is a suitable measure of disease activity in cystic fibrosis
- ○ B is used to assess lung function of pre-school children
- ○ C is increased in asthma
- ○ D represents the volume of air expired in 1 second during a forced expiratory manoeuvre
- ○ E can indicate large and medium airway obstruction

7. An enlarged tongue is a typical feature of

- ○ A hypothyroidism
- ○ B trisomy 18
- ○ C Pierre Robin sequence
- ○ D GM1 gangliosidosis
- ○ E neurofibromatosis type 1

8. Causes of bronchiectasis include

- ○ A sarcoidosis
- ○ B primary ciliary dyskinesia
- ○ C gastro-oesophageal reflux
- ○ D pertussis infection
- ○ E measles infection

9. In early lung development

- ○ A the airways and parenchyma are derived from mesoderm
- ○ B pulmonary surfactant production begins at 24/40
- ○ C alveolar development is complete at term
- ○ D surfactant reduces alveolar surface tension
- ○ E thyroid hormone inhibits surfactant production

10. Adrenaline (epinephrine)

- ○ A is secreted from the adrenal cortex
- ○ B stimulates β_2 receptors
- ○ C should be used by the intravenous route in anaphylaxis
- ○ D causes hypoglycaemia
- ○ E causes dilatation of renal vasculature

11. The following is true of food allergy

○ A peanuts are the commonest cause of fatal food-induced reactions
○ B allergy to hen's egg is commonly outgrown
○ C other allergies are uncommon
○ D the diagnosis can be made on the history alone
○ E peanut allergy usually resolves

12. The following is true of of tuberculosis

○ A the incidence is falling worldwide
○ B notification to public health authorities is required
○ C a tuberculin test wheal > 5 mm is significant in any child
○ D isoniazid can cause peripheral neuropathy
○ E children are less prone to extra-pulmonary complications than adults

13. In cystic fibrosis

○ A life expectancy depends upon nutritional status
○ B life expectancy is, on average, 20 years
○ C eczema can cause a false-positive sweat test
○ D cystic fibrosis transmembrane conductance regulator (CFTR) fails to absorb chloride ions in the lungs
○ E raised *Aspergillus* IgG titre is characteristic of allergic bronchopulmonary aspergillosis

14. The following cause vasoconstriction of the pulmonary circulation

○ A hypoxia
○ B nitric oxide
○ C prostaglandin I_2
○ D platelet activating factor
○ E histamine

15. Lung compliance in infants

○ A is defined as the volume change per unit of pressure
○ B increases with age
○ C is increased in respiratory distress syndrome
○ D is independent of lung volume
○ E is dependent on type II pneumocytes

16. Recognised extrapulmonary complications of cystic fibrosis include

○ A hypertrophic osteoarthopathy
○ B rectal prolapse
○ C glomerulonephritis
○ D azoospermia
○ E diabetes mellitus

questions

17. Recognised associations of primary ciliary dyskinesia include
- ○ A infertility
- ○ B nasal polyps
- ○ C hydrocephalus
- ○ D bronchiectasis
- ○ E malabsorption

18. Differential diagnoses of bronchiolitis in infants includes
- ○ A total anomalous pulmonary venous drainage
- ○ B pertussis infection
- ○ C gastro-oesophageal reflux
- ○ D interstitial pneumonitis
- ○ E pneumococcal pneumonia

Best of Five Questions

19. Parents come to you for antenatal counselling; the mother is a carrier of a cystic fibrosis mutation and the father has never been tested and has no family history. Which ONE of the following is the chance that their offspring may have cystic fibrosis?

○ A 1 in 4
○ B 1 in 100
○ C 1 in 160
○ D 1 in 200
○ E 1 in 2500

20. A 2-year-old boy has a history of lethargy and falling asleep during the day. His mother reports that he snores loudly. Which is the MOST useful investigation?

○ A Arterial blood gas
○ B Electrocardiogram (ECG)
○ C Microlaryngobronchoscopy (MLB)
○ D Overnight oxygen saturation recording
○ E Lateral upper airways X-ray

21. A 14-month-old girl with a history of eczema develops generalised urticaria, wheeze and severe dyspnoea shortly after eating some peanut butter for the first time. What is the MOST appropriate initial treatment?

○ A Adrenaline intramuscularly
○ B Adrenaline intravenously
○ C Hydrocortisone intravenously
○ D Chlorpheniramine intravenously
○ E Chlorpheniramine orally

22. In an 8-year-old boy with inspiratory stridor due to compression of the trachea, what would you MOST expect the spirometry flow–volume loop to show limitation of?

○ A Peak expiratory flow rate (PEF)
○ B Forced expiratory flow rate (FEF$_{25-75}$)
○ C Expiratory flow only
○ D Inspiratory flow only
○ E Inspiratory and expiratory flow

23. A 10-year-old boy who was previously well presents with a 2-week history of malaise and headache, with pleuritic chest pain, cough and fever over the past 3 days. Five days of treatment with oral penicillin has made no improvement. On examination there is a small area of stony dullness at the right lung base. The MOST likely diagnosis is which of the following?

- ○ A Lymphoma
- ○ B *Mycoplasma pneumoniae* pneumonia
- ○ C Pneumococcal pneumonia
- ○ D *Pneumocystis carinii* pneumonia
- ○ E Staphylococcal pneumonia

24. In a child who presents with ascending paralysis of the legs and areflexia, what is the MOST useful method of respiratory monitoring?

- ○ A Respiratory rate
- ○ B Partial pressure of carbon dioxide in arterial blood (Pco_2)
- ○ C Oxygen saturation
- ○ D Vital capacity
- ○ E Peak expiratory flow rate

25. A 3-month-old baby has a history of wheeze and coughing usually after feeds, since birth. Her weight is normal and on examination she has a Harrison sulcus and a hyper-expanded chest. Which of the following investigations would be the MOST useful?

- ○ A Flexible bronchoscopy
- ○ B Computed tomography (CT) scan of the chest
- ○ C Ciliary brushing for motility
- ○ D Sweat electrolytes
- ○ E Upper gastrointestinal (GI) contrast study

26. An 18-month-old girl presents with a 6-month history of weight loss and cough. Examination reveals a clear chest, cervical lymphadenopathy and red, tender lesions on her shins. Which is the MOST useful diagnostic test?

- ○ A Erythrocyte sedimentation rate (ESR)
- ○ B Bronchoalveolar lavage
- ○ C Sputum culture
- ○ D Gastric aspirate
- ○ E Skin biopsy

27. A 10-year-old boy presents to your general paediatric clinic with a long history of asthma. It is poorly controlled and he suffers frequent exacerbations. Which one of the following measures of lung function would be MOST useful?

○ A Total lung capacity (TLC)
○ B Serial peak expiratory flow (PEF) rates
○ C Transfer factor
○ D FEF_{25-75}
○ E Residual volume

Extended Matching Questions

28. Theme: Causes of chest disease

A   Bronchopulmonary dysplasia
B   Acute lymphoblastic leukaemia
C   Asthma
D   Interstitial pneumonitis
E   Cystic fibrosis
F   Rheumatoid lung disease
G   Pulmonary tuberculosis
H   Allergic bronchopulmonary aspergillosis
I   Primary ciliary dyskinesia

For each of the following case scenarios select the most likely diagnosis from the list above. Each option may be used once, more than once, or not at all.

○   1. A 6-year-old boy has a history of failure to thrive and multiple chest infections. On examination he has digital clubbing and coarse crackles throughout his chest. Haemoglobin: 11.2 g/dL. Forced expiratory volume in 1 second (FEV_1): 86% of expected. Chest X-ray (CXR): Bilateral streaky shadowing.

○   2. An 11-year-old girl presents with a persistent cough. Over the past 6 weeks her weight centile has fallen from the 9th to < 0.4th. On examination she has digital clubbing and unilateral monophonic wheeze. Haemoglobin: 8.2 g/dL. FEV_1: 90% of expected. CXR: unilateral peri-hilar shadowing.

○   3. A 2-year-old boy has a history of failure to thrive, multiple chest infections, perennial rhinitis and chronic secretory otitis media. On examination he has a blocked nose, digital clubbing, and bilateral coarse crackles are audible throughout his chest. Haemoglobin: 12.5 g/dL. CXR: Bilateral streaky shadowing, dextrocardia.

29. Theme: Investigation of children with respiratory disease

A   Sputum bacteriology
B   Nasal brushing
C   Bronchoalveolar lavage
D   Lateral neck X-ray
E   Barium swallow
F   Rigid bronchoscopy
G   Serum *Aspergillus* specific IgE
H   Flow–volume loop
I   Serum viral studies

For each of the following case scenarios select the most useful investigation from the list above. Each option may be used once, more than once, or not at all.

○ 1. A 10-year-old boy with cystic fibrosis has a history of persistent wheeze and breathlessness. His symptoms require daily oral prednisolone for control. Chest X-ray (CXR): bilateral patchy upper lobe shadows. Forced expiratory volume in 1 second (FEV$_1$): 65% of expected. Serum IgE: > 5000 IU/L.

○ 2. A 2-year-old boy presents with a 2-day history of a persistent dry cough. On examination he has right-sided monophonic wheeze. CXR: hyper-luscent right lung, liver displaced downwards.

○ 3. A 5-month-old girl with HIV infection presents with a 1-week history of fever, cough and dyspnoea. On examination there are crackles throughout her chest. Oxygen saturation: 85%. CXR: bilateral diffuse shadowing. Nasopharyngeal aspirate for bacteria, viruses and fungi: normal.

30. Theme: Outpatient management of children with asthma

A Referral to a respiratory paediatrician
B Inhaled beclometasone dipropionate 400 μg per day
C Leukotriene receptor antagonist
D Inhaled short-acting β$_2$-agonist as required
E No change
F Inhaled beclometasone dipropionate 800 μg per day
G Slow-release oral theophylline
H Long-acting β$_2$-agonist (LABA)

For each of the following scenarios select the most appropriate possible addition or change to outpatient management from the list above. Each option may be used once, more than once, or not at all.

○ 1. A 5-year-old boy with asthma regularly uses inhaled beclometasone dipropionate at a dose of 200 μg per day. He finds that that he still wakes up with wheeze every morning and needs to use his β$_2$-agonist inhaler daily.

○ 2. A 9-year-old girl with asthma is reviewed after 3 months. She has been taking 800 μg of inhaled beclometasone dipropionate per day, a long-acting β2-agonist and a short-acting β2-agonist as required. She reports that her symptoms have improved greatly and she now hardly uses her short-acting β2-agonist.

○ 3. A 3-year-old boy with asthma has persistently poor control despite regular use of inhaled beclometasone dipropionate 400 μg /day.

answers

1. Erythema nodosum

Answers: A C D

Erythema nodosum are tender, nodular erythematous lesions which occur most commonly on the shins followed by thighs and arms. They last for 1–2 months and evolve into blue bruise-like lesions. Causes include infections (*Streptococcus*, *Salmonella*, *Yersinia*, *Campylobacter*, tuberculosis, *Chlamydia*, hepatitis B, and Epstein–Barr virus), inflammatory disorders (such as sarcoidosis, ulcerative colitis and Crohn's disease), malignancy and drugs, sulphonamides and the oral contraceptive pill.

2. Oxyhaemoglobin dissociation curve

Answers: A D

Haemoglobin (Hb) affinity for oxygen increases as the partial pressure of oxygen in arterial blood increases. This is shown as a sigmoid-shaped plot of Hb saturation against partial pressure of oxygen (the oxy-Hb dissociation curve). The flat upper portion allows arterial oxygen content to stay high despite variations in P_{O_2}. The steep middle portion of the curve describes how peripheral tissues (with a lower partial pressure of oxygen) can withdraw large amounts of oxygen from Hb for only a small drop in capillary P_{O_2}. A variety of conditions can alter the binding affinity of Hb for oxygen, thus shifting the curve left or right. Increases in temperature, carbon dioxide partial pressure, hydrogen ion concentration, and D-2,3-diphosphoglycerate all shift the curve to the right, facilitating oxygen removal from the blood by peripheral tissues, as the affinity of Hb for oxygen decreases. Opposite changes and fetal Hb result in a left-shifted curve.

3. Gas transfer across alveolar capillary membrane

Answers: B C E

The exchange of gas at the alveolar–capillary interface is achieved by passive diffusion. Fick's Law states that the diffusion of gas is proportional to the tissue area of the membrane and the difference between the partial pressures of the gases on opposite sides. Diffusion is inversely proportional to the thickness of the membrane. Properties of the gas are also important, diffusion is proportional to gas solubility and inversely proportional to the square root of its molecular weight. Carbon dioxide diffuses through tissues 20 times faster than oxygen, because it is more soluble. According to Fick's Law, the volume of gas transferred is given by:

$$V_{gas} = \frac{\{A \times D \times (P_1-P_2)\}}{T}$$

where A = membrane area, T = membrane thickness, D = diffusion constant, P_1-P_2 = difference in partial pressures.

4. Digital clubbing

Answers: A D E

Digital clubbing is an important clinical sign. The first change is loss of the nail-fold angle and a fluctuant bogginess of the nail bed. Increased curvature of the nail bed and enlargement of the distal phalanx occur later. Causes include any cause of bronchiectasis or cyanotic heart disease, tuberculosis, empyema, malignancy, bacterial endocarditis, biliary cirrhosis, chronic active hepatitis and inflammatory bowel disease.

5. Nasal polyps

Answers: B C D

Nasal polyps present with nasal obstruction, symptoms of rhinitis (decreased smell and rhinorrhoea) and an enlarged nasal bridge. Very often they are ignored, as they can present insidiously. Cystic fibrosis must be considered in any child with nasal polyps, but they also occur in chronic rhinitis and the triad of nasal polyps, asthma and aspirin hypersensitivity (Sampter's triad), more commonly seen in older children and adults. Wegener's granulomatosis is a necrotising vasculitis found in the lungs, joints, eyes, kidneys, sinuses and nasopharynx. It causes ulceration and bony destruction in the nose, with symptoms of rhinorrhoea, nasal congestion and sinus pain.

6. Percentage of predicted FEV$_1$

Answers: A D E

Lung function testing in preschool children is limited to research centres. From 5 years of age most children can perform spirometry, with practice. FEV$_1$ represents the volume of air expired in 1 second during a forced expiratory manoeuvre and gives an indication of large and medium airway diameter. Results are calculated as a percentage of expected results for a healthy child of similar age, height, age and sex. It is the best measure of lung function for children with cystic fibrosis and when measured over time it can indicate prognosis. In obstructive airway diseases such as asthma, the FEV$_1$ and ratio of FEV$_1$ to forced vital capacity (FVC) are reduced, showing baseline airway obstruction. An improvement in FEV$_1$ of at least 15% after administration of an inhaled bronchodilator is indicative of asthma. Bronchial challenge tests can also be used in the diagnosis of asthma; administration of methacholine causes a 20% fall in FEV$_1$ for 3 hours.

7. Enlarged tongue

Answers: A C D

An enlarged tongue can obstruct the airway and lead to an emergency, particularly in infants who have small nasal passages. Tongue-reduction surgery is successful. It occurs in hypothyroidism, mucopolysaccharidoses, trisomy 21 and Beckwith–Wiedemann syndrome. Pierre Robin sequence is caused by a posterior attachment of the tongue together with a small mandible resulting in pseudo-macroglossia and the tongue commonly falls back to obstruct the airway.

8. Causes of bronchiectasis

Answer: All true

Bronchiectasis arises where there is permanent dilatation of the sub-segmental airways associated with inflammation. Accumulation of exudative material in the dilated airways leads to the clinical manifestation of copious muco-purulent sputum production. Poor appetite and weight gain are also common. Examination reveals clubbing and coarse crackles throughout the chest. There are many causes including cystic fibrosis, immunoglobulin deficiency, and primary ciliary dyskinesia. Pertussis and measles were historically important causes, reduced in incidence by immunisation. Treatment involves elimination of respiratory infection (vigorous treatment of acute infections and colonisation), effective mucous clearance (physiotherapy with or without mucolytic drugs) and increased calorie intake.

9. Early lung development

Answers: B D

Early lung development starts with a ventral out pouching of the fore-gut, lined by endodermal epithelium. This gives rise to right and left lung buds which by 6 weeks contain segmental bronchi. By 16 weeks all the conducting airways are present, as blind tubes lined by cuboidal epithelium (pseudo-glandular stage). Cilia and cartilage begin to develop. From 17–24 weeks (canalicular stage) distal airway epithelium thins out in preparation for gas exchange. The lungs become vascularised and surfactant synthesis begins. In the alveolar sac stage (25–40 weeks) thin-walled saccules at the end of respiratory bronchioles develop into alveoli. After birth, the majority of lung development occurs in the respiratory unit and alveoli continue to be formed until approximately 3–8 years, when the number of alveoli reaches that of an adult. Surfactant is a mixture of surface-active phospholipids which reduce alveolar membrane surface tension, reducing the negative pressure the infant needs to generate to expand alveoli. Surfactant production is increased by glucocorticoids and thyroid hormone.

10. Adrenaline

Answer: B

Adrenaline is an endogenous catecholamine secreted by the adrenal medulla. With increasing dose it stimulates β_1 (increased heart rate and contractility) and β_2 receptors (bronchodilatation, peripheral vasodilatation and reflex tachycardia). At higher doses α-receptor stimulation dominates, causing peripheral vasoconstriction and elevation of systolic blood pressure. Adrenaline inhibits insulin release, causing hyperglycaemia. Adrenaline is the treatment of choice for severe allergic reactions (anaphylaxis) and should only be administered intramuscularly, except in extreme circumstances. Children who have had a previous allergic reaction involving airway narrowing or who also have asthma should be provided with pre-loaded adrenaline syringes.

11. Food allergy

Answers: A B

The perceived prevalence of food allergy is high (20%) but the prevalence of confirmed food allergy is more likely to be 2–3% in children. Nearly all food allergic children have suffered from some other allergy, such as eczema or asthma or less commonly rhinitis. Egg and milk allergies are usually outgrown by school age, with more severe cases persisting. Peanut allergy on the other hand is longer lasting and it will resolve in only 20% of those with mild allergy. Again, more severe cases are likely to be long lived. Diagnosis is made on the basis of a typical history of an allergic reaction occurring soon after ingestion of a likely allergen. This is confirmed by detection of specific IgE to the allergen either by skin prick test, or in the serum (CAP-RAST test). In equivocal cases oral challenge may be used. Treatment involves providing detailed written and verbal avoidance advice, together with a written emergency treatment plan detailing how and when to give oral antihistamine and/or intramuscular adrenaline.

12. Tuberculosis

Answers: B D

The incidence of tuberculosis worldwide is rising reflecting increasing HIV (human immunodeficiency virus) infection, poverty and overcrowding. All cases must be reported to public health authorities. The lungs are the commonest site of infection and source of spread, although extrapulmonary complications, like tuberculous meningitis, are more common among children than adults. Symptoms are highly variable so one must always consider the diagnosis in any child who presents with fever, anorexia, weight loss and cough. Therapy is with isoniazid and rifampicin for 6 months and pyrazinamide for 2 months. Rifampicin turns secretions, such as tears (warn patients not to wear contact lenses) and urine orange. Isoniazid and rifampicin can cause deranged liver function tests and isoniazid can cause peripheral neuropathy. Ethambutol (risk of visual disturbance) is used in resistant or high-risk cases.

answers

13. Cystic fibrosis

Answers: A C

Cystic fibrosis is an inherited recessive disorder of chloride secretion in the lungs and exocrine glands. The gene on chromosome 7 encodes CFTR. Deficiencies in CFTR lead to failure of chloride ion secretion and excessive sodium ion absorption, leading to dehydration of airway secretions. The ions are transported in the opposite direction in sweat glands and this forms the basis for the sweat test; a sodium or chloride ion concentration > 60 mEq/L is diagnostic. Median life expectancy is now 40 years. Allergic bronchopulmonary aspergillosis (ABPA) occurs in cystic fibrosis and asthma. It results from an overzealous IgE host response to colonisation with *Aspergillus*. Typical findings are wheeze and a dry cough. Patchy infiltrates on CXR appear in different sites over time; a high total and *Aspergillus* specific IgE together with *Aspergillus* precipitins help with the diagnosis. Treatment is with oral corticosteroids and anti-fungal agents (eg itraconazole).

14. Vasoconstriction of pulmonary circulation

Answers: A D E

The pulmonary circulation delivers blood to the alveoli for gas exchange. The relatively low mean pulmonary arterial pressure (15 mmHg) is maintained even though the pulmonary arteries receive the entire cardiac output, because of the extremely low vascular resistance. If the cardiac output increases (eg in exercise) then the low resistance system will dilate and recruit previously closed vessels, to accommodate. However, pulmonary vessels can also be made to constrict, and one of the most powerful stimuli is hypoxia (diverting circulation away from under-ventilated areas thus avoiding ventilation/perfusion mismatch). Nitric oxide is a powerful vasodilator which can be administered via inspired gas to treat pulmonary hypertension. Platelet aggregating factor and histamine are released during inflammatory and allergic reactions respectively causing vasoconstriction.

15. Lung compliance

Answers: A B E

Lung compliance is defined as the change in lung volume per unit of pressure. It is also represented by the slope of the pressure–volume curve. This is a sigmoid shape, so compliance also depends on the initial lung volume, from which the change in volume was measured (eg at large lung volumes where the lung is near its elastic limit, the pressure–volume curve is less steep and hence compliance is reduced). Pulmonary surfactant produced by type II pneumocytes in newborns reduces surface tension and increases compliance. In respiratory distress syndrome there is a deficiency of surfactant (most commonly due to prematurity) and compliance is reduced.

16. Complications of cystic fibrosis

Answers: A B D E

There are many extrapulmonary complications of cystic fibrosis (CF). Gastrointestinal complications include pancreatic insufficiency (causing steatorrhoea and weight loss) and diabetes mellitus (due to pancreatic fibrosis). Diabetes in CF is often straightforward to control and ketoacidosis is uncommon. Diabetes gets more common with age affecting 7% of adults with CF. Meconium ileus in the neonatal period occurs in 15% of patients with CF and distal intestinal obstruction syndrome (DIOS) in 10%. The diagnosis should be considered in children who present with rectal prolapse, although constipation is a more common cause of this condition. Approximately 98% of men with CF are infertile due to vas deferens obstruction. Sex hormone function is normal but puberty is commonly delayed due to malnutrition. Treatment of infections with aminoglycoside antibiotics over time can damage renal tubules.

17. Primary ciliary dyskinesia

Answers: A B C D

Primary ciliary dyskinesia occurs in one in 15, 000 births, with autosomal recessive inheritance. It results in abnormalities of cilia such as missing dynein arms, absence of radial spokes or aplasia. In the respiratory tract this results in failure of the mucociliary elevator and clearance of secretions, leading to bronchiectasis, chronic rhinitis and glue ear. Fifty percent also have dextrocardia and situs inversus (Kartagener's syndrome). Infertility through impaired sperm motility and hydrocephalus, presumably due to impaired ventricular ependymal cilia, also occur. Diagnosis is suggested by low exhaled nitric oxide and confirmed by nasal brushing for ciliary beat frequency and electron microscopy. Treatment is with physiotherapy and antibiotics with specialist Ear Nose and Throat (ENT) assessment.

18. Bronchiolitis in infants

Answer: All true

Bronchiolitis is an acute respiratory infection, most commonly caused by a respiratory syncytial virus (RSV). The symptoms and signs are respiratory distress and coryza, hyperinflation, occasionally apnoea and widespread crackles on auscultation. Many conditions can mimic bronchiolitis and one should be particularly aware of the possibility of cardiac lesion. Treatment is supportive with oxygen, clearance of secretions and hydration as appropriate. Infants with bronchopulmonary dysplasia may benefit from a humanised monoclonal anti-RSV antibody (palivizumab).

19. B: 1 in 100

This question illustrates the commonly examined topic of inheritance. You will be expected to know the carrier frequency (1/25) and the prevalence in the general population of cystic fibrosis (1/2500) and other common conditions. We know the mother is a carrier and the father has a 1/25 chance of being a carrier so the calculation $1 \times 1/25 \times 1/4 = 1/100$ gives the odds per pregnancy of producing a child with cystic fibrosis. The abnormal gene codes for cystic fibrosis transmembrane conductance regulator (CFTR), whose main role is as an ATP-dependent chloride ion channel. Defects in CFTR in the lung result in reduced chloride secretion and hyperabsorption of sodium ions leading to viscid secretions. Remember that CFTR works in reverse in the skin leading to failure to reabsorb sweat and hence high sweat electrolytes – the basis of the sweat test.

20. D: Overnight oxygen saturation recording

This child has a history suggestive of sleep apnoea. The presentation can be subtle and families will often not report pauses in breathing whilst asleep unless specifically questioned. Other features which are suggestive are early morning headaches (due to high arterial CO_2 partial pressure (Pco_2) and an 'adenoidal' voice. It is most often caused by adenotonsillar hypertrophy but neuromuscular conditions must also be considered. Arterial blood gas may show high Pco_2 and upper airway XR or MLB may reveal large adenoids, but most information will be obtained from overnight oxygen saturation monitoring. This will detect periods of desaturation and apnoea, and linked to analysis of chest and abdominal movements can help distinguish between obstructive causes (tonsils) and central causes (eg brain stem tumour).

21. A: Adrenaline intramuscularly

The history clearly describes an episode of anaphylaxis. Adrenaline is the most important single drug in anaphylaxis. It reverses upper and lower airway oedema, causes bronchodilation, increases blood pressure and causes peripheral vasoconstriction, reducing capillary leak. It should be given by the intramuscular route in most cases. The intravenous route should only be used by those experienced in this method and at a concentration of no greater than 1 in 10,000, with ECG monitoring. The prevalence of peanut allergy in childhood has tripled over the past decade and it now affects 1.5%. Up to 80% of children with peanut allergy react on the first apparent ingestion, suggesting prior occult sensitisation. The median age at onset is 2 years and only 20% of young children with mild allergy can expect to grow out of it. A management plan for nut-allergic children which includes avoidance advice and a tailored patient-held self-treatment plan, together with regular follow up, can reduce the number of further nut-induced reactions. Future potential treatments include use of anti-IgE and desensitisation with modified peanut allergen.

22. D: Inspiratory flow only

Examination of the spirometry trace is important, in addition to interpretation of values such as FEV_1. We can deduce that the lesion is causing a dynamic obstruction as there are only symptoms on inspiration; fixed lesions cause obstruction in both inspiration and expiration. A dynamic extra-thoracic obstruction causes limitation of inspiratory flow only. Dynamic intra-thoracic airway obstruction, as occurs in asthma, causes reduction of expiratory flow and therefore FEV_1 and FEF_{25-75}.

23. B: *Mycoplasma pneumoniae* pneumonia

Mycoplasma pneumoniae is a common cause of atypical pneumonia among school-age children. The clues in the history are malaise and headache, more common in *Mycoplasma* infection, together with the age of the child and lack of responsiveness to penicillin (*Mycoplasma* lack a cell wall). Macrolide antibiotics are the treatment of choice. *Pneumocystis carinii* infection usually only affects children with a severe underlying immune deficiency, such as HIV, severe combined immunodeficiency syndrome (SCID), di George syndrome, and post bone-marrow transplantation (BMT).

24. D: Vital capacity

The case scenario describes Guillain–Barré syndrome, a post-inflammatory infectious polyneuropathy. However, regardless of the cause all neurological conditions which affect breathing need careful monitoring because deterioration and respiratory failure can be clinically silent. Peak expiratory flow rate will be normal until very late; the best measure is vital capacity. Also pay attention to bulbar function because failure of gag and cough reflexes leave the patient vulnerable to aspiration and possible asphyxiation.

25. E: Upper gastrointestinal (GI) contrast study

This child presents with a picture of lower airway obstruction that is associated with feeds, implying the presence of gastro-oesophageal reflux disease, an H-type tracheo-oesophageal fistula (TOF) or viral-induced wheeze. The most useful information would come from an upper GI contrast study which should include a tube oesophogram to exclude a TOF. Flexible bronchoscopy is poor for excluding TOF, and ciliary brushing is used only for the diagnosis of primary ciliary dyskinesia. It would be sensible to screen for cystic fibrosis at a later stage.

26. D: Gastric aspirate

The scenario describes a child with tuberculosis, the red lesions suggesting erythema nodosum. The presentation can be subtle with few chest signs. The classic features of fever, lethargy and weight loss can be absent in children. Acid-fast bacilli are best obtained by gastric washings, usually on three successive mornings; bronchoalveolar lavage has a lower yield. The diagnosis can be confirmed by intradermal tuberculin testing. Initial treatment consists of isoniazid (for 6 months), rifampicin (6 months) and pyrazinamide (2 months). Monitor liver function tests and examine for peripheral neuropathy.

27. B: Peak expiratory flow (PEF) rate

Lung function testing can be useful in asthma. Serial measurements of peak expiratory flow rate are easy to perform and are suitable for home monitoring. It is the most useful measure available to a general paediatrician. Total lung capacity and residual volume both increase in asthma, representing air-trapping by obstructed airways. The ideal measure of small airway function is FEF $_{25-75}$. It represents forced expiratory flow between 25% and 75% of vital capacity and is less effort-dependent, but is only available with spirometry. Transfer factor measures diffusion of carbon monoxide and gives an estimate of lung diffusion capacity (reduced in consolidation and fibrosis and increased in pulmonary haemorrhage).

28. CAUSES OF CHEST DISEASE

1. E – Cystic fibrosis

This is a typical presentation of bronchiectasis with failure to thrive, a history of chest infections, and digital clubbing. Possible causes from the list of options are cystic fibrosis and primary ciliary dyskinesia of which cystic fibrosis is more prevalent (1 in 2500 versus 1 in 15, 000) and therefore the most likely diagnosis. Further clues that the diagnosis is cystic fibrosis may include a history suggestive of malabsorption (pancreatic insufficiency) or sub-acute bowel obstruction (distal intestinal obstruction syndrome), meconium ileus, rectal prolapse, chest infections with staphylococcus as an infant, or with pseudomonas at school age. Liver dysfunction leading to hepatosplenomegaly may also be apparent.

2. G – Pulmonary tuberculosis

The girl presents with anaemia, weight loss and monophonic wheeze, with a CXR suggestive of hilar lymphadenopathy. Two possible diagnoses are pulmonary tuberculosis (TB) and haematological malignancy. The presence of digital clubbing makes pulmonary TB a more likely diagnosis.

3. I – Primary ciliary dyskinesia

This case is very similar to case (1). However there is a predominance of upper airway symptoms which makes primary ciliary dyskinesia the most likely diagnosis. Other clues may include a family history of male infertility (autosomal recessive inheritance), dextrocardia in 50%, and abdominal situs inversus. Treatment is as for cystic fibrosis with the addition of specialist Ear, Nose and Throat (ENT) management.

29. INVESTIGATION OF CHILDREN WITH RESPIRATORY DISEASE

1. G – Serum *Aspergillus* specific IgE

Allergic bronchopulmonary aspergillosis is a recognised complication of cystic fibrosis and less commonly asthma. It arises as an overzealous allergic reaction to *Aspergillus* colonisation within the airways, leading to mucous impaction and airway narrowing, particularly of the upper lobes. Patients present with dry cough, wheeze and deterioration of lung function tests. It is suspected if total serum IgE is very high and *Aspergillus* specific IgE and *Aspergillus* precipitins are raised. Treatment is with long courses of oral steroids and anti-fungal agents such as itraconazole.

2. F – Rigid bronchoscopy

Foreign-body aspiration must always be considered in children who present with a monophonic wheeze and unilateral hyper-expansion on X-ray. Rigid bronchoscopy is suitable for removal of such objects – flexible bronchoscopes are too narrow.

3. C – Bronchoalveolar lavage

The girl is likely to have *Pneumocystis carinii* pneumonia. This extracellular parasite causes a relatively common opportunistic infection in patients with T lymphocyte immunodeficiencies (eg HIV infection, CD40 ligand deficiency, or Di George syndrome). Peak incidence is at age 3–6 months. Even when hypoxia is present, chest auscultation may reveal no crackles. CXR almost always shows bilateral diffuse alveolar shadowing. Bronchoalveolar lavage is the best method for isolating the organism, if it cannot be isolated from nasopharyngeal aspirate (NPA) or sputum. Treatment is with high-dose trimethoprim–sulfamethoxazole, pentamidine, or dapsone. Children at risk of infection should receive prophylactic trimethoprim–sulfamethoxazole.

30. OUTPATIENT MANAGEMENT OF CHILDREN WITH ASTHMA

1. H – Long-acting β_2-agonist (LABA)

New guidelines on the management of asthma were published by the British Thoracic Society (*Thorax* 2003 **58**(Suppl 1):i1–i83. website – http://thorax.bmjjournals.com/content/vol58/suppl_1). The aims are to control symptoms, prevent exacerbations, achieve the best possible lung function and minimise side effects. The principles are to achieve early control and maintain it by increasing and decreasing therapy as necessary, usually at 3-month intervals. The next option for the boy is to add a LABA and assess his response.

2. B – Inhaled beclometasone dipropionate 400 µg per day

This case illustrates that stepping-down treatment should be considered every 3 months, to minimise side effects from steroids.

3. C – Leukotriene receptor antagonist

A change to the updated British Thoracic Society guidelines was the inclusion of leukotriene receptor antagonists in children aged 2–5 years who have poor control despite maximal steroid therapy.

Rheumatology

Nathan Hasson

Multiple Choice Questions

1. The following are characteristic features of juvenile idiopathic arthritis

- A the majority of patients are positive for rheumatoid factor
- B arthritis is present for a minimum of 3 months
- C it only occurs in children under 16 years of age
- D it occurs in 1 in 1000 children
- E it is more frequent in girls

2. The following is true of systemic onset juvenile idiopathic arthritis

- A it usually occurs in children under 5 years of age
- B fevers last for more than 2 weeks
- C only cervical lymphadenopathy is seen
- D antinuclear antibody is usually positive
- E disseminated intravascular coagulation is a recognised complication

3. In polyarticular juvenile idiopathic arthritis

- A rheumatoid factor is occasionally positive
- B low-grade fever is common
- C thrombocytosis is seen
- D methotrexate is the treatment of choice
- E three joints or more are affected

4. The following is true of oligoarticular juvenile idiopathic arthritis

- A it is more common in females
- B antinuclear antibody is usually positive
- C methotrexate is the treatment of choice
- D the affected limb has decelerated growth
- E it is usually seen after the age of 8 years

5. Juvenile psoriatic arthritis is associated with

- ○ A skin rash
- ○ B nail pitting
- ○ C antinuclear antibody positivity
- ○ D family history of psoriasis
- ○ E a poor response to methotrexate

6. In arthritis associated with inflammatory bowel disease

- ○ A disease course is usually polyarticular
- ○ B erythema nodosum is a recognised association
- ○ C human leukocyte antigen HLA B27 is present
- ○ D sulfasalazine is the drug of choice
- ○ E poor outcome of the joint disease is usual

7. Juvenile dermatomyositis is associated with

- ○ A a rash in a malar distribution
- ○ B a rash over the extensor surfaces of fingers
- ○ C nasal speech
- ○ D antinuclear antibody positivity in the majority
- ○ E raised serum levels of lactate dehydrogenase

8. Features of systemic lupus erythematosus include

- ○ A oral ulceration
- ○ B photosensitivity
- ○ C lymphopenia
- ○ D inflammatory bowel disease
- ○ E rheumatoid factor positivity

9. Characteristic features of Henoch–Schönlein purpura include

- ○ A onset before 3 years of age
- ○ B flitting arthritis
- ○ C minor abdominal pain
- ○ D immunoglobulin A complexes in affected skin on biopsy
- ○ E good response to methotrexate

10. Kawasaki disease is associated with

- ○ A fever for at least 5 days
- ○ B purulent conjunctivitis
- ○ C thrombocytopenia
- ○ D coronary artery aneurysms in 30%
- ○ E generalized lymphadenopathy

11. Recognised features of Wegener's granulomatosis are

- A destructive granulomata in the sinuses
- B skin rash
- C positive antineutrophilic cytoplasm antibody
- D pulmonary lesions
- E good response to methotrexate

12. The following are features of polyarteritis nodosa

- A fever
- B abdominal pain
- C low white cell count
- D steroids are contraindicated
- E *Staphylococcus* is a recognised trigger

13. The following are associated with rheumatic fever

- A group A streptococcal infection
- B subcutaneous nodules
- C antinuclear antibody positive
- D arthralgia
- E erythema multiforme

14. Causes of antinuclear antibody positivity in children include

- A systemic lupus erythematosus
- B systemic onset juvenile idiopathic arthritis
- C Parvovirus infection
- D scleroderma
- E mixed connective tissue disease

15. The following are side effects of methotrexate

- A nausea
- B pulmonary fibrosis
- C transaminitis
- D raised platelets
- E rash

Best of Five Questions

16. A 3-year-old girl presents with a 3-week history of fever, with daily spikes of 40°C, a pink rash that varies, painful muscles, some swelling of her wrists for 7 weeks, and generalized lymphadenopathy. Investigations reveal anaemia, with a high white cell count, raised platelets, very high erythrocyte sedimentation rate and C reactive protein. Antinuclear antibody, double-stranded DNA, and rheumatoid factor are negative. Which of the following is the MOST likely diagnosis?

- ○ A Systemic lupus erythematosus
- ○ B Acute lymphoblastic leukaemia
- ○ C Systemic onset juvenile idiopathic arthritis
- ○ D Parvovirus infection
- ○ E Neuroblastoma

17. A 5-year-old boy presents with a 2-month history of rash around his eyes, an inability to brush his hair, nasal speech, and he uses Gower's manoeuvre to get up from the floor. His creatine kinase is normal but his lactate dehydrogenase is raised. What is the MOST likely diagnosis?

- ○ A Becker muscular dystrophy
- ○ B Systemic lupus erythematosus
- ○ C Juvenile dermatomyositis
- ○ D Myasthenia gravis
- ○ E Viral myositis

18. An 8-year-old boy presents with an 8-week history of swelling of both knees, and a dry rash over his elbows and knees. His father has dry skin patches in his scalp. He also is found to have swelling of two of his toes. His GP has been treating him for a fungal infection of his nails. What is the MOST likely diagnosis?

- ○ A Enthesitis-related juvenile idiopathic arthritis
- ○ B Psoriatic arthritis
- ○ C Oligoarticular juvenile idiopathic arthritis
- ○ D Juvenile dermatomyositis
- ○ E Inflammatory bowel disease related arthritis

19. A 5-year-old boy presents with a history of recurrent right knee pain for 4 weeks. He has had difficulty with sport, and now he limps. Previously he was very active, and was very good at gymnastics. He had two bouts of tonsillitis recently, neither of which required antibiotic treatment. There has been no fever or rash. Examination reveals a completely normal right knee and the only abnormality is loss of internal rotation at the right hip, but no pain. What is the MOST likely diagnosis?

- ○ A Oligoarticular juvenile idiopathic arthritis
- ○ B Benign joint hypermobility syndrome
- ○ C Enthesitis-related arthritis
- ○ D Perthes disease
- ○ E Reactive arthritis

Extended Matching Question

20. Theme: Rheumatology case studies

A   Systemic onset juvenile idiopathic arthritis
B   Polyarticular juvenile idiopathic arthritis
C   Oligoarticular juvenile idiopathic arthritis
D   Enthesitis related arthritis
E   Psoriatic arthritis
F   Systemic lupus erythematosus
G   Juvenile dermatomyositis
H   Acute lymphoblastic leukaemia
I   Chronic fatigue syndrome
J   Polyarteritis nodosa

For each of the following case scenarios select the most likely diagnosis from those listed above. Each option may be used once, more than once, or not at all.

○ 1. A 4-year-old boy presents with a 1-month history of fever, rash, and painful joints. On examination he has arthritis in both knees but the rest of his joints are clinically normal. He has rash on his face. Investigations show (normal ranges in brackets): haemoglobin 6.5 g/dL (10.5–12.5); white cell count 5.6 (5–15) (lymphocytes 0.7); platelets 100 (150–400); erythrocyte sedimentation rate 67 mm/h (< 15); C reactive protein 4 (< 7); antinuclear antibody 1 in 2560; bone marrow blasts 1% (0–2%).

○ 2. A 9-year-old boy presents with pain in both heels for 3 months. He has also been to the GP with a painful red eye on several occasions. On examination he has an effusion in his left knee, decreased range of movement in his right hip, and tenderness along the Achilles tendons and heel. His erythrocyte sedimentation rate was 100 mm/h; C reactive protein 45 (< 7); full blood count normal; human leukocyte antigen (HLA) B27 positive.

○ 3. A 5-year-old girl presents with arthritis in her right knee and left wrist for 2 months. She has generalised lymphadenopathy. Ophthalmological examination is normal. Investigations show her antinuclear antibody is negative. Her erythrocyte sedimentation rate is 65 mm/h; C reactive protein 40 (< 7); full blood count shows a haemoglobin of 9 g/dL (10.5–12.5); white cell count 2.3 (5–15); platelets 97 (150–400).

answers

1. Juvenile idiopathic arthritis

Answers: D E

The new classification of 'juvenile idiopathic arthritis' replaces the old one of 'juvenile chronic/rheumatoid arthritis'. Most patients are negative for rheumatoid factor; with only 2–3% positive. For diagnosis of juvenile idiopathic arthritis, arthritis has to be present for 6 weeks rather than the old criterion of 3 months, in a patient aged less than 16 years. Systemic onset juvenile idiopathic arthritis also occurs in adults. Incidence is 1 in 1000 and there are eight subtypes. Generally more girls are seen, as the oligoarticular form is the commonest, which is more frequent in girls.

2. Systemic onset juvenile idiopathic arthritis

Answers: A B E

Systemic onset is more common in children aged less than 5 years old. Incidence is equal in boys and girls. The definition is a minimum of 2 weeks of fevers, in which daily spikes are seen. The rash is a fleeting salmon-pink colour. Generalised lymphadenopathy is seen – unlike in Kawasaki disease, where only cervical adenopathy is a diagnostic criteria. Antinuclear antibody and rheumatoid factor are usually negative. Disseminated intravascular coagulation is occasionally seen as a complication.

3. Polyarticular juvenile idiopathic arthritis

Answers: A C D

Rheumatoid factor is positive in 2–3% of polyarticular juvenile idiopathic arthritis patients. Low-grade fevers are only occasionally seen. Thrombocytosis is a feature, as are raised erythrocyte sedimentation rate and C reactive protein. Methotrexate is the drug of choice in both positive rheumatoid factor and negative rheumatoid factor polyarticular juvenile idiopathic arthritis. Five joints or more are affected.

4. Oligoarticular juvenile idiopathic arthritis

Answers: A B

Oligoarticular juvenile idiopathic arthritis is the commonest subtype of juvenile idiopathic arthritis. It is diagnosed if four joints or less are affected in the first 6 months of the disease. Oligoarticular juvenile idiopathic arthritis is four times more common in females. Antinuclear antibody is positive in 60–70% of patients. Methotrexate is rarely used to treat the disease except for non-responsive disease or severe anterior uveitis. The affected limb – especially if a knee is affected – has accelerated growth. It is usually seen under the age of 6 years. It is termed persistent oligo-juvenile idiopathic arthritis if arthritis is restricted to four joints or less after the first 6 months of disease, and extended oligo-juvenile idiopathic arthritis if more than four joints are affected after the first 6 months of disease.

5. Juvenile psoriatic arthritis

Answers: A B C D

In psoriatic arthritis the rash may or may not be coincident with arthritis. Nail pitting is seen in psoriasis. Dactylitis of fingers or toes is seen and is typical. Distal interphalangeal joint arthritis is also typical. It can affect a few or many joints. Some patients may develop uveitis so slit-lamp monitoring is needed. Some patients are positive for antinuclear antibody, and have a family history of psoriasis. The condition responds well to methotrexate.

6. Arthritis associated with inflammatory bowel disease

Answers: B C D

Inflammatory bowel disease-related arthritis is usually oligoarticular in course. Several different skin lesions including erythema nodosum are seen. HLA B27 positivity is a feature. Sulfasalazine is the disease-modifying drug of choice. Good joint outcome is usually seen.

7. Juvenile dermatomyositis

Answers: B C E

Rash is usually around the eyes, associated with oedema, and spares the malar area. Gottron's papules occur on the extensor surfaces of fingers, and are red raised papular lesions. Palatal weakness leads to nasal speech. Antinuclear antibody is only positive in a small percentage. Creatine kinase levels can be normal but lactate dehydrogenase is often raised.

8. Systemic lupus erythematosus

Answers: All true

These are all features of systemic lupus erythematosus. The 1997 American College of Rheumatology criteria include most of these. Renal disease is fairly common in children with systemic lupus erythematosus. A person shall be said to have systemic lupus erythematosus if any four or more of the following 11 criteria are present:
1. Malar rash
2. Discoid rash
3. Photosensitivity
4. Oral ulcers
5. Non-erosive arthritis of more than one joint

6. Serositis (pleuritis; or pericarditis)
7. Renal disorder (persistent proteinuria > 0.5 g/day; or cellular casts)
8. Neurological disorder (seizures; or psychosis)
9. Haematological disorder (haemolytic anaemia; or leukopenia; or lymphopenia; or thrombocytopenia)
10. Immunological disorder (anti-phospholipid antibodies; or anti-DNA antibody to native DNA; or anti-Sm antibody to Sm nuclear; or false-positive serological test for syphilis)
11. Antinuclear antibody (abnormal titre).

9. Henoch–Schönlein purpura

Answers: D

Henoch–Schönlein purpura usually occurs after the age of 3 years. There is a male predominance. The arthritis is very painful but is not flitting, as in rheumatic fever. Abdominal pain is usually severe, and complications such as intussusception occur. Immunoglobulin A complexes are seen in the skin and glomeruli if biopsied. Renal involvement is common. Non-steroidal anti-inflammatory drugs are used, and occasionally steroids, to manage the arthritis – but not methotrexate.

10. Kawasaki disease

Answers: A

Five days of fever is necessary for the diagnosis. The conjunctiva is red but not purulent. Thrombocytosis is seen rather than thrombocytopenia. Aneurysms of the coronary artery and other large arteries are seen in 20%. Cervical (rather than generalized) lymphadenopathy only is a diagnostic criteria. Erythema of palms and soles with oedema and subsequent peeling are seen. Erythema of the lips with oral inflammation are also part of the diagnostic criteria.

11. Wegener's granulomatosis

Answers: A B C D

Wegener's is a granulomatous vasculitic disease. Biopsies of affected tissues show granulomas. Destructive granulomata occur in the ears, the nose and the sinuses. Rash, pulmonary and renal lesions are seen. Antineutrophilic cytoplasmic antibodies are positive in Wegener's. The treatment is steroids and cyclophosphamide for systemic disease.

12. Polyarteritis nodosa

Answers: A B

Polyarteritis nodosa is a vasculitis affecting small to medium sized muscular arteries. Polyarteritis nodosa can present with fever and abdominal pain. Leucocytosis is a feature. Treatment is usually with high-dose steroids.

Streptococcal infection – rather than staphylococcal infection – is a trigger, so antistreptolysin O test should be performed and penicillin prophylaxis used. Aneurysms are diagnosed by angiography and are present in small to medium-sized muscular arteries such as renal, liver, splenic end bowel.

13. Rheumatic fever

Answers: A B D

For the diagnosis there has to be proof of group A streptococcal infection. Subcutaneous nodules are a major criterion. You must have two major criteria or one major and two minor criteria for the diagnosis. Antinuclear antibody is usually negative. Arthralgia is quite often severe, and is a minor criterion. The classical rash is erythema marginatum, which is a major criterion. The revised Jones' criteria include the following major manifestations:

- Carditis
- Polyarthritis
- Erythema marginatum
- Subcutaneous nodules
- Chorea

The revised Jones' criteria include the following minor manifestations:

- Fever
- Arthralgia
- Previous rheumatic fever or rheumatic heart disease
- Raised erythrocyte sedimentation rate or C reactive protein
- Prolonged PR interval on ECG.

14. Antinuclear antibody positivity

Answers: A D E

Of patients with systemic lupus erythematous, 97% are positive for antinuclear antibody. Systemic onset juvenile idiopathic arthritis is not associated with antinuclear antibody. Ebstein–Barr viral infection – not parvovirus – is associated with antinuclear antibody. In both scleroderma and mixed connective tissue disease patients are often antinuclear antibody positive. Causes of antinuclear antibody positivity in children include:

- Systemic lupus erythematosus
- Juvenile idiopathic arthritis
- Chronic active hepatitis
- Scleroderma
- Mixed connective tissue disease
- Drugs (eg anticonvulsants)
- Ebstein–Barr virus infection.

15. Side effects of methotrexate

Answers: A C

Methotrexate is the most frequently used disease-modifying drug in paediatric rheumatology. It is not only used in juvenile idiopathic arthritis, but also in dermatomyositis, scleroderma, and in some patients with lupus. It can cause nausea which responds to anti-emetics such as odansetron, or nausea can be avoided if administered by subcutaneous injection. It can cause mouth ulcers, and folic acid supplements are given to prevent this and other side effects. Pulmonary fibrosis is said to occur in adults but is not seen in paediatric practice. Liver enzymes can rise, but not usually resulting in liver fibrosis. It can lower platelet or white cell counts, and occasionally haemoglobin. Rash is not usually a side effect.

16. C: Systemic onset juvenile idiopathic arthritis

These are all the classical findings in systemic onset juvenile idiopathic arthritis. More than a 2-week history of spiking fevers is one of the criteria needed for the diagnosis. The rash is salmon pink and can vary in intensity over the day, being prominent at times of fever. Generalised lymphadenopathy is a common feature. Arthritis has to be present for more than 6 weeks in systemic onset juvenile idiopathic arthritis. Systemic lupus erythematosus usually has a positive antinuclear antibody and normal C reactive protein. Platelets are usually normal or low in acute lymphoblastic leukaemia. The history is too prolonged for parvovirus, and rash is unusual in neuroblastoma, as is high platelet count.

17. C: Juvenile dermatomyositis

The features are all classical of juvenile dermatomyositis. The rash around the eyes is the violaceous heliotrope seen in juvenile dermatomyositis. The weakness is proximal and more often worse in the upper limbs. Palatal weakness causes nasal speech. Quite often creatine kinase can be normal but lactate dehydrogenase raised. In Becker muscular dystrophy the creatine kinase is very high. There are not enough features for the diagnosis of lupus erythematosus. Myasthenia gravis is not associated with rash. Viral myositis often affects the calf muscles and has an associated high creatine kinase.

18. B: Psoriatic arthritis

Psoriatic arthritis can present with few or several joints affected. It can occur without the classical psoriatic rash but occasionally a psoriatic-like rash as described here can be seen. Dactylitis is a feature of psoriatic arthritis and is rarely seen in other types of juvenile idiopathic arthritis. The father's dry scalp patches may possibly be psoriatic and family history is often seen. The nail problem may be psoriatic and typically pitting is seen. In enthesitis-related arthritis, enthesitis and tendonitis are features – which are not seen in this patient. Enthesitis is inflammation at the site of tendon insertion into bones such as the posterior heel.

19. D: Perthes disease

Perthes disease is avascular necrosis of the femoral head. It is more common in boys of this age. Frequently it presents with referred pain to the knee, rather than hip pain. The only sign on examination may be loss of internal rotation initially. There can be an associated synovitis. The history is too short for oligoarticular juvenile idiopathic arthritis (6 weeks being necessary for the diagnosis) and the hip is almost never affected with this. The patient is probably hypermobile given that he is good at gymnastics, but the range of movement would be increased with often 90° of internal rotation, rather than the limited movement of this patient. The history is possible for reactive arthritis, but an irritable hip would not last for 4 weeks, and it is unusual in other reactive arthritides for the hip to be affected.

20. RHEUMATOLOGY CASE STUDIES

1. F – Systemic lupus erythematosus

These are all typical of systemic lupus erythematosus and there are enough features to fulfil the diagnostic criteria.

2. D – Enthesitis-related arthritis

These are all the features of enthesitis-related arthritis.

3. H – Acute lymphoblastic leukaemia

This girl is unlikely to have oligoarticular juvenile idiopathic arthritis with these blood results, because the erythrocyte sedimentation rate and C reactive protein level are not usually raised, and the full blood count is very abnormal. In particular the platelets are low.

Statistics

Angie Wade

Multiple Choice Questions

1. Randomisation of patients to treatments within a trial ensures that

○ A the patient is unaware of the treatment group to which they are assigned

○ B each patient has an equal chance of being in any treatment group

○ C the treatment group is known before consent is obtained

○ D although individuals receive different treatments, each patient will be allocated to the treatment most likely to benefit them

○ E differences between treatments will be significant

2. Within a clinical trial, allocation of patients to treatments should, where possible, be

○ A blinded

○ B randomised

○ C systematic

○ D decided prior to obtaining consent

○ E performed away from the study centre

3. In a trial of vitamin supplementation on reaction times among 12-year-olds, which of the following need to occur for 'social class' to be a confounder?

○ A reaction times are different in the supplemented and non-supplemented (control) groups

○ B the children are not randomised to treatment groups

○ C the supplemented group have a different social class distribution to the non-supplemented (control) group

○ D the non-supplemented (control) group are all children of professional parents

○ E reaction times are associated with social class

4. A new asthma inhaler is tested against a standard inhaler within a double-blind crossover trial. With this study design

- A neither the patient nor the assessor knows which treatment (standard or new) is being given at any time
- B any differences found between the new and standard inhaler must be significant
- C the order of treatments (new and standard) should be randomised
- D fewer patients will be needed than if a parallel trial of new versus standard inhalers had been used
- E the outcome must be normally distributed

5. Observational studies

- A cannot be randomised
- B give more convincing evidence of true differences than experimental studies
- C are always large
- D can never be useful
- E must be blinded

6. The following is true when age-matched and sex-matched pairs of patients are allocated to new or standard treatments

- A age and sex cannot confound the study results
- B randomisation to the new or standard treatment should take place within pairs
- C the treatment allocations must be blinded
- D the pairing should be retained in the analysis
- E disease severity will be similar between the treatment groups

7. The following are categoric variables

- A height
- B social class
- C age
- D gender
- E ethnicity

8. When data are ranked

- A the highest rank is equal to the total number in the sample
- B the median is the middle ranked value
- C the lowest value has rank 1
- D any equal data values must be removed from the sample prior to ranking
- E the mean of the values is the middle-ranked value

9. **An oxygenation index is measured in a group of 30 children aged less than 10 years. The values obtained range from 2 to 250, the median value is 27, and the mean is 60. In this situation**

- ○ A the distribution of the oxygenation measurements is upwardly skew
- ○ B the best average value to use is the mean
- ○ C the mean is heavily influenced by relatively few children with high oxygenation values
- ○ D this oxygenation index is not a reliable measurement
- ○ E more measurements need to be made

10. **One hundred 12-year-old children with fragile X syndrome undergo intelligence testing. Their mean IQ is 97 (standard deviation 5). The measurements are approximately normally distributed. In this study**

- ○ A the standard error of the measurements is 0.5 IQ points
- ○ B a 95% confidence interval for the population mean IQ of 12-year-old with fragile X is (96, 98) based on this sample
- ○ C approximately 95% of the children have IQ measurements in the range 87 to 107
- ○ D the mean IQ in this sample is significantly different from the expected mean of 100 amongst normal children
- ○ E the distribution of IQ is skew

11. **The standard error of an estimate**

- ○ A is smaller for larger sample sizes
- ○ B is a measure of the precision of that estimate
- ○ C cannot be negative
- ○ D depends on the average value of the sample
- ○ E is used to construct confidence intervals

12. **A p value**

- ○ A indicates the statistical significance of any differences seen in the sample(s)
- ○ B lies between -1 and $+1$
- ○ C is more useful than a confidence interval for interpreting results
- ○ D is the probability of obtaining the current sample if the null hypothesis is true
- ○ E indicates the clinical significance of any differences seen in the sample(s)

13. **A parametric correlation coefficient**

- ○ A must be positive
- ○ B of zero indicates no relationship between the measurements
- ○ C takes the value 1 only if the points lie on the line of equality
- ○ D shows the extent to which two continuous measurements are linearly related
- ○ E is negative if there is no association

14. **Reflex times are measured in a group of children aged 5 to 15 years old. The correlation between reflex time and age is calculated as 0.76 (95% confidence interval 0.7, 0.82). In this study**

○ A the correlation coefficient is significantly different to zero
○ B more measurements need to be made
○ C there is a linear association between reflex times and age
○ D the association is clinically important
○ E older children tend to have slower reflex times

15. **In a group of asthmatic children there is a tendency for heavier children to have lower lung functions. It is true that**

○ A losing weight will improve lung function
○ B weight affects lung function
○ C the correlation between weight and lung function will be negative
○ D social class may be a confounder
○ E there needs to be a control group to compare these values with

16. **The following statistics associated with screening tests are directly dependent on prevalence**

○ A sensitivity
○ B specificity
○ C likelihood ratio
○ D positive predictive value
○ E proportion of false positives

17. **An ultrasound screen is applied to 500 pregnant women at risk of Down syndrome based on their age and previous medical history. Seventy fetuses are found to have femur lengths in the upper decile of the normal distribution. Of these 70 fetuses, 25 with extreme measurements had Down syndrome – as opposed to only 30 of the fetuses with measurements not in the upper decile. In this analysis, the following is true**

○ A the specificity of the test as a screen for Down syndrome is 45/445
○ B 25/70 is the positive predictive value of the test (measurement in the upper decile)
○ C the sensitivity of femur length in the upper decile for diagnosing Down syndrome is 30/55
○ D of those with measurements in the upper decile most will not have Down syndrome
○ E the study shows that age is an important predictor of Down syndrome

18. **Blood pressure is measured in two groups of people. Those receiving some treatment have blood pressures that are on average 6 mmHg lower than those in the untreated group. A t-test was applied and $p = 0.02$, 95% confidence interval for the difference (4.16, 7.84) mmHg. It is true to say that**

○ A the treatment should be introduced as it may be clinically relevant
○ B the treatment must have improved blood pressure by at least 4.16 mmHg on average in the population
○ C the difference observed would have occurred by chance 1 time in 20 if there really was no treatment effect
○ D randomisation to groups was not successful
○ E the t-test would not have been appropriate if the blood pressure measurements were skew

19. **The number of children positive for a certain genetic defect were compared across groups of asthmatic children and healthy controls of a similar age. It can be said that**

○ A the study is invalid because it is not randomised
○ B a t-test could be used to assess the significance of the differences between groups
○ C chi-square could be used to test the significance of the differences in proportions that were positive in the two groups
○ D age may be a confounder
○ E a confidence interval for the difference in proportions that were positive would help to interpret the results

20. **The power of a study**

○ A varies between -1 and $+1$
○ B can be calculated retrospectively
○ C is the probability of correctly rejecting the null hypothesis when it is false
○ D increases as the sample size is increased
○ E is larger the greater the difference that is to be detected

21. **Within a randomised controlled trial, of 100 individuals who received standard care, 40 had an adverse event in the following year. This is in contrast to 20 of 100 who received a programme of intensified care. It is true that**

○ A the percentage reduction in adverse events attributable to intensified care is 20%
○ B the number that need to be treated (NNT) to avoid 1 adverse event is 5
○ C relative risk (RR) is 0.5
○ D a confidence interval for the percentage reduction will depend on the sample size
○ E age may be a confounder in the comparison

Best of Five Questions

22. **In children with renal failure, a study shows that vitamin D levels are found to be severely depleted ($p < 0.0001$). Which is the MOST appropriate course of action based on this study?**
    - A Introduce vitamin D supplementation as standard practice
    - B Consider extent of depletion, clinical implications, costs of supplementation and make a decision based on these
    - C Re-analyse the data taking into account the ages of the children
    - D Carry out a further study of greater size
    - E Do nothing

23. **Cirrhotic children aged 6–10 years old are randomised to a new dietary regimen or standard advice. After 2 years their height standard deviation (sd) scores are compared. The group allocated to the new diet have a higher mean sd score for height (difference 0.2, 95% confidence interval (–0.8, 1.2)) but this difference is non-significant ($p = 0.52$). An improvement of 0.2 sd scores over a 2-year period would be considered clinically important in this group of children. Which is the MOST appropriate course of action based on this study?**
    - A Do nothing further – the study has shown the new diet is not statistically significantly better than current practice
    - B Re-analyse the data using non-parametric methods
    - C Follow the children for longer to try and obtain statistical as well as clinical significance
    - D Carry out a trial of a larger size to obtain a more precise estimate of the effect of the new diet compared to standard
    - E Introduce the new diet as standard practice – the average improvement is clinically important

24. **Haemoglobin measurements were made in small groups of children with five different syndromes. In order to assess whether there are differences between the groups that are unlikely to have occurred by chance, which one of the following is MOST appropriate?**
    - A A further study of much larger size
    - B Analysis of variance comparing means between the groups
    - C The data should be plotted according to syndromic group
    - D Mann–Whitney U-tests between each pair of syndromic groups
    - E Non-parametric analysis of variance comparing medians between groups (Kruskal–Wallis)

questions

25. **What is the BEST reason why concurrent control groups are useful when performing studies?**

○ A They allow the use of statistical tests for the comparison of two groups (eg two sample t-tests)
○ B They help to ensure that any differences seen are due to the treatment or disease being studied
○ C They allow the study to be blinded
○ D They help boost the overall numbers studied
○ E They are better than historical controls

26. **Which of the following applies MOST to a reference range for CD4 counts in childhood?**

○ A The study should be based on large numbers of children
○ B The study needs to be age-related
○ C It is useful for assessing children with known disease
○ D It allows the CD4 counts of individual children to be compared to what is expected for normal children of that age
○ E It does not give the sensitivity of low CD4 count in detecting disease

27. **Intelligence (IQ) assessments and heights are measured in a group of healthy 7-year-olds. To investigate whether there is a meaningful statistically significant relationship which of the following is MOST appropriate?**

○ A The correlation coefficient should be calculated
○ B A regression analysis should be used and the regression coefficient presented with confidence interval
○ C A p value must be obtained
○ D More assessments could be made
○ E Heights should be expressed as sd (standard deviation) scores

Extended Matching Questions

28. Theme: Significance tests

A   Two sample t-test
B   Paired t-test
C   Mann–Whitney U-test
D   One-way analysis of variance
E   Kruskal–Wallis analysis of variance
F   Regression analysis
G   Correlation coefficient
H   Chi-square

For each of the following study scenarios choose the most appropriate statistical test from the list above to analyse the data. Each option may be used once, more than once, or not at all.

○ 1. Blood pressure measurements are made in a group of children with pituitary hormone disorders and age- and sex-matched control pairs. The study aims to investigate whether pituitary hormone disorders are associated with altered blood pressure.

○ 2. Developmental tests are applied to determine whether children who were admitted to intensive care in the neonatal period are more likely to have delayed development at age 5 than those who were not.

○ 3. Blood pressures (assumed normally distributed) are compared between 5-year-olds from four different clearly defined racial backgrounds

29. Theme: Interpreting trial results

A   The difference is statistically and clinically significant; the new cream should not be introduced
B   The difference is statistically significant but difference is clinically small; the new cream should be introduced
C   A larger study is required to determine whether it is worth introducing the new cream
D   The difference between the creams is both statistically and clinically significant; the new cream should be introduced
E   The difference is statistically significant but the difference is not of clinical importance and the new cream should not be introduced
F   The study provides enough evidence to discount the usefulness of the new cream
H   The study is invalidated by the drop-outs
I   The results cannot be interpreted because the analysis used was inappropriate

A randomised controlled trial is used to compare the effectiveness of a new cream (T) for treating eczema compared to the current alternative cream (C) for children aged 5–10 years of age. Severity is rated on a 0 (no rash) to 10 (severe

rash) scale. An average fall of 2 points on the severity scale attributable to the new cream would be deemed of clinical importance and worth changing to the new cream to achieve. For the following study results choose the most appropriate interpretation from the list above. Each option may be used once, more than once, or not at all.

○ 1. Those allocated to the new cream have an average rating of 5.4 compared with 7.8 for those on the current alternative (95% confidence interval for the difference $(-3.6, -1.2)$, $p < 0.0005$).

○ 2. Those allocated to the new cream have an average rating of 5.4 compared with 7.8 for those on the current alternative (95% confidence interval for the difference $(-6.0, 1.2)$, $p = 0.23$).

○ 3. Of the 40 children allocated to the two creams, 30 who used the new cream had an average severity rating of 5.4. The 50 children who used the current treatment (40 randomised to this treatment plus the 10 who did not use the new cream but reverted to current) had an average rating of 7.8. The 95% confidence interval for the mean fall in severity rating (-2.4) was $(-2.6, -1.2)$, $p < 0.0005$.

30. Theme: Diagnostic testing

A   Sensitivity
B   Specificity
C   Positive predictive value
D   Negative predictive value
E   False-positive rate
F   False-negative rate
G   Positive likelihood ratio
H   Negative likelihood ratio
I   Percentage correctly classified
J   The prevalence of miscarriage

During the first trimester of pregnancy, 400 women at high risk of miscarriage have ultrasound measurements of nuchal fold thickness. Subsequently, 80 of these women miscarry. 100 women had abnormal nuchal fold values.

Considering abnormal nuchal fold thickness as a potential diagnostic test for miscarriage in this group, which of the above items has a value of 75%? Each option may be used once, more than once, or not at all.

○ 1. Equal numbers of those that miscarry have abnormal or normal nuchal fold thickness.

○ 2. Of those who subsequently miscarry, 75 have abnormal nuchal fold thickness.

○ 3. Of those with abnormal nuchal fold thicknesses, 60 subsequently miscarry.

answers

1. Randomisation to treatments in a trial

Answer: B

Participants should be randomised to groups to remove any potential bias, meaning that each patient has the same chance of being assigned to either of the groups, regardless of their personal characteristics. Randomisation aims to ensure that the treatment groups are similar apart from the treatment under study, hence any differences in outcome are more easily attributable to being causally related to treatment. It is the procedure of blinding – not randomisation – that ensures that individuals do not know which groups they are in. Randomisation should take place after consent is obtained. Randomisation does not ensure that differences in treatments will be significant.

2. Allocation of patients to treatments

Answers: A B E

Allocation to treatments should be random rather than systematic to avoid potential bias. Ideally randomisation should be made via telephone, so that the process cannot be influenced by any known features of the patient. Consent should be obtained before treatment group is determined otherwise the approach taken to gaining consent (and/or the patient's decision to consent or not) may be affected by the planned allocation. If the patient and/or the clinician (or assessor) know which treatment a patient is having, then this may influence their recorded outcome. A study is blind when either the patient and/or the clinician (assessor) does not know the treatment allocation. Single blind is the term used when one of the two (patient or clinician/assessor) does not know the allocation but the other does. Double blind means that neither knows about it.

3. Social class as a confounder

Answers: C E

A confounding factor is a background variable (something not of direct interest) that is distributed differently between the groups being compared, and which affects the outcome being studied. So for social class to be a confounder in the comparison of reaction times between those supplemented and those who are not, the social class distribution must differ between supplemented and non-supplemented groups and social class must affect reaction times.

4. Double-blind crossover trial of asthma inhaler

Answers: A C D

In a crossover study, each patient receives treatment and placebo in a random order. Fewer patients are needed because many between-patient confounders may be removed. The order of treatments should be randomised, otherwise bias may be introduced if there is an order effect. A study is double blind if neither the patient nor the researcher assessing the patients (or the treating clinician) knows which treatment the patient has been randomised to receive. The outcome may or may not be normally distributed. Choosing a particular study design (crossover) does not make the outcome normally distributed. Any differences found in outcome during the two treatment periods may or may not be statistically significant and/or clinically significant. There may be differences that are non-significant.

5. Observational studies

Answer: A

In observational studies the groups being compared are already defined and the study merely observes what happens. Since groups (different diseases or different treatments) are already determined and known they cannot be blind or randomised. The size of the sample that is studied is determined by the researcher and may be small. If a difference is found in an observational study then it is more likely to be due to confounding factors than it is in an experimental trial, because the groups were determined before the study. A difference found with an experimental design is more likely to result from the treatment than it is in an observational study. Despite the potential for confounding, observational studies can provide useful information. Interpretation of the results should take into account the limitations of the design.

6. Age-matched and sex-matched pairs

Answers: A B D

Confounding may be avoided by matching individuals in the groups according to potential confounders. Here, individuals of the same age and sex are allocated to new or standard treatments within pairs. Therefore the new and standard groups will have the same age and sex distribution and these two variables cannot be confounders. Randomisation to new or standard treatment should take place within the pair and this pairing should be retained in the analysis. Ideally treatment allocation should be blinded, but it may not be possible to do so for these particular treatments. All individuals of the same age and sex are not necessarily similar in their disease severity, hence matching for age and sex does not ensure that disease severity will be similar between the groups.

7. Categoric variables

Answers: B D E

Data may be either categoric or numeric. With categoric variables, each individual lies in one category. Numeric data are measured on a number scale. Height and age are both numeric. Social class falls into one of five or six categories depending on how it is defined. Gender is only either male or female (one of two categories) and ethnicity may be divided into a variable number of categories.

8. Ranked data

Answers: A B C

Ranks give the order of increasing magnitude of numeric variables. The lowest value has rank 1. The highest value will have a rank equal to the total number in the sample (if there are 10 values, then the ranks 1 to 10 will be assigned and the largest value will have rank 10). Half of the values will be smaller than the middle ranked value and half will be larger, hence the middle-ranked value is the median (50th centile). If the data are skew then the mean and median will be different, and because the median is always the middle-ranked value the mean will not be equal to the middle-ranked value if the data are skew . Equal data values should be given equal ranks. To achieve this, the corresponding ranks will be averaged between the data values. Each value in the dataset should be given a rank. Data values that are the same do not need to (should not) be removed from the sample prior to ranking.

9. Oxygenation index in children

Answers: A C

For symmetrically distributed data, the mean and median values are the same and will be mid-way between the extreme values of the distribution. When data are skew then the mean is pulled in the direction of the skew, away from the median. Skew is named according to the direction of the outlying tail. For the oxygenation index, the mean is larger than the median and both are much closer to the lowest value of 2 than to the highest value of 250. Hence it is reasonable to assume that most individuals have relatively low oxygenation values and there are a few with high values that have a large influence on the mean (making it much larger than the median). The mean is influenced by a few large values, so it is not representative of the bulk of the values – the median is a much better measure of what is average or representative of most individuals. No measure of the precision of the estimates of mean and median are given. The precision will depend on the sample size. Hence the group of 30 children may or may not give adequate information – we would need to estimate the precision and see whether this is suitable for our needs. If greater precision is required then a larger sample would have to be taken. Reliability is the extent to which the measurements would be replicated if taken again (eg at a different time or by a different assessor). The values given are based on a single measurement in each child and this gives us no information about reliability.

10. Intelligence tests in fragile X syndrome

Answers: A B C D

Normally distributed data are symmetric and therefore not skew. Since the measurements are approximately normally distributed, then we would expect about 95% of them to lie within a range mean ± 2 standard deviations (97 ± 2(5) = 97 ± 10 = 87, 107). The standard error is calculated as the standard deviation divided by the square root of the sample size and the interval (mean ± 2 standard errors) is an approximate 95% confidence interval for the population mean. Hence, for this sample, standard error = $5/\sqrt(100) = 5/10 = 0.5$ and a 95% confidence interval is given by (97 ± 2(0.5)) = (97 ± 1) = (96, 98). The confidence interval gives the range of population values that the sample data are compatible with. In this case the interval (96, 98) excludes the expected mean of 100 found amongst normal children. Hence the mean IQ in the sample is significantly different from 100.

11. Standard error of an estimate

Answers: A B C E

The standard error is a measure of how precisely the sample value approximates the true population value. For continuous data it is calculated as the standard deviation divided by the square root of the sample size. Confidence intervals can be constructed around the sample estimate using the standard error. Precision will obviously be greater or better for larger sample sizes and we can also see this from the formula for calculating standard error. (The standard deviation is divided by the square root of the sample size, hence as the sample size increases we divide by a larger number, and the standard error will be smaller, indicating greater or better precision.) Also, since the standard deviation is always positive, the standard error must also be positive. Although it depends on the spread of the values around the average (ie the standard deviation) it does not depend on the average itself, being a measure of the precision of that average.

12. *p* value

Answers: A D

The *p* value is the probability of obtaining the current sample if the null hypothesis were true. It gives a measure of the statistical significance of any differences seen. As it is a probability it can range from 0 (no probability/never happens) to 1 (certainty/always happens) but cannot be negative. The *p* value gives an indication of how likely one particular hypothesised value is to be true, whereas the confidence interval gives the range of hypothesised values

answers

with which the sample is compatible. Hence confidence intervals give much more information and enable clinical interpretation of the results. The p value gives statistical significance, but clinical significance will depend on other factors such as inconvenience associated with treatment, level of improvement, or difference and costs.

13. Parametric correlation coefficient

Answer: D

The most commonly used correlation coefficient is Pearson's, which is parametric. It gives a measure of the linear association between two continuous measurements. Non-parametric correlation coefficients (Spearman or Kendall) measure the tendency for one variable to fall or rise as the other increases – whether this tendency is linear or not. All correlation coefficients can take values between –1 and +1. Negative values indicate that as one of the variables increases the other decreases. A value of 1 indicates a perfect positive relationship, and if the correlation coefficient is parametric then this would mean that the points lie on a straight line (however the line is not necessarily the line of equality). A Pearson correlation coefficient of zero (0) indicates that there is no linear association between the variables, although there may still be a non-linear one.

14. Reflex times

Answers: A C

The correlation coefficient gives a measure of linear association between reflex times and age. Zero indicates no linear association, the closer the value is to +1 or –1, the stronger the linear association. For this sample, the value is 0.76, which indicates some linear association. The coefficient is positive and this shows that age and reflex time both increase together (that is, older children have longer reflex times). The confidence interval for the correlation (0.7, 0.82) does not contain zero and the correlation is therefore significantly different to zero. Whether or not more measurements need to be made depends on whether the precision obtained for the estimate is suitable for whatever purpose it was made. The association is statistically significant, whether it is clinically important depends on additional factors.

15. Lung function in heavier asthmatic children

Answers: C D

If heavier children have lower lung functions then as weight increases lung function will tend to decrease, so the correlation between these two variables will be negative. This is an observational study and measurements are only made once on each child. Hence, whilst there is a relationship between the variables, there is no evidence that if individual children change their weight that this will result in a change of lung function. The relationship observed between weight and lung function may be due to some other factor that may be causally related to lung function, and which acts as a confounder. For example, if the children from lower social classes tend to be heavier, and low social class adversely influences lung function (maybe due to a genetic component or behavioural factors) then indeed social class will be a confounder in the comparison. To study the relationship between weight and lung function among asthmatic children, a selection of asthmatic children with differing weights only is required and a further comparison group is not necessary.

16. Prevalence-dependent statistics

Answers: D E

The prevalence of a disease is the proportion of the population with the disease. The sensitivity of a screening test is the proportion of those with disease who screen positive. Therefore, because it is based solely on those with disease, this does not vary if the prevalence changes. The specificity is the proportion of those without the disease who screen negative. Therefore, because it is based solely on those without disease, it does not vary if the prevalence changes. The likelihood ratio can be calculated from the sensitivity and specificity and because these are not prevalence dependent, the likelihood ratio will not be either. The positive predictive value is the proportion of those who screen positive who actually have the disease. In a population with low prevalence, most will not have disease and for a given specificity the proportion of false positives in the population will be quite high and this will make the positive predictive value tend to be lower (less of those screening positive do have disease). Conversely, if the prevalence is high then the proportion of false positives will be relatively low (the number of non-diseased people are lower, so the number of misdiagnosed people are also lower) and the positive predictive value will tend to be higher.

17. Screen for risk of Down syndrome

Answers: B D

We need to construct a 2 × 2 table of screen test results against true diagnosis. This is the information as given.

PPL in upper decile	Down syndrome		Total
	Yes	No	
Yes	25		70
No	30		
Total			500

And the rest can be completed from this information. Note: check that all the marginal totals agree before proceeding (eg 70 + 430 = 500; 55 + 445 = 500).

PPL in upper decile	Down syndrome		
	Yes	No	Total
Yes	25	45	70
No	30	400	430
Total	55	445	500

The specificity is the proportion of those without disease who screen negatively, thus 400/445 (A is false). The positive predictive value is the proportion of those who screen positive who actually have disease (25/70). The sensitivity of the test is the proportion of those with Down syndrome who test positive (25/55). Of the 70 fetuses with measurements in the upper decile, most (45) do not have Down syndrome. The study gives no information about the relationship between age and Down syndrome.

18. Treatment for blood pressure

Answer: E

The difference observed is statistically significant and would have occurred by chance 2 times in 100 (since $p = 0.02$) or 1 time in 50 if there really were no treatment effect. We cannot tell from the information given whether or not randomisation was successful. The sample is compatible with average fall in blood pressure of between 4.16 and 7.84 mmHg. We are 95% confident that the population average fall lies within this interval, however it may not (in fact, 5% of the time it will not). Statistical significance does not necessarily imply clinical significance or relevance. The *t*-test is not valid if the measurements are not normally distributed. Skew data are not normally distributed.

19. Genetic defect in asthmatic and healthy children

Answers: C E

This is an observational study and cannot be randomised. We cannot allocate asthma randomly. For a variable to be a confounder it must differ between the groups being compared and it must also affect outcome. Since the asthmatic and healthy children are of similar ages, age cannot be a confounder in the comparison. Presenting the difference in proportions positive in the two groups, together with a confidence interval to show the precision with which this difference is estimated, would be informative. *t*-Tests are appropriate for continuous numeric outcomes. Chi-square can be used to compare differences in proportions.

20. Power of a study

Answers: B C D E

The power of a study is the probability (usually expressed as a percentage) of correctly rejecting the null hypothesis when it is false. As it is a probability it must lie between 0 and 1 (or 0 and 100% when expressed as percentage). The greater the difference to be detected, the greater the chance that the study will find it; hence the power is larger for bigger differences. The larger the sample size, the greater the power to detect a difference of a given size. Power is usually calculated at the commencement of a study. Sample size is often based on achieving a given power to detect differences of clinically important magnitude. Sample size estimation is based on unknown quantities and the estimations of power may be made once those quantities have been determined from the sample data. Hence power may be calculated retrospectively.

21. Adverse events in randomised controlled trial

Answer: All true

The percentage suffering from an adverse event fell from 40% to 20%, hence the reduction was 20%. With a 20% fall this means that an extra five individuals would need to receive intensified care for one to avoid an adverse event. Hence the number needed to treat (NNT) is 5. A confidence interval around the percentage reduction (20%) will take into account the sample size – the greater the sample size the more precise the estimate of the difference attributable to intensified care and the narrower the confidence interval. The relative risk is given by: the risk in the intensified care group divided by the risk in the standard care group (20 ÷ 40 = 0.5). If the groups (standard and intensified care) differ in their age distribution and age affects outcome (adverse event yes/no) then age would be a confounder in the comparison.

22. B: Consider extent of depletion, clinical implications, costs of supplementation and make a decision based on these

There is a statistically significant difference as shown by the *p* value. We are not told who the renal failure children are compared with to get that value. Was this concurrent healthy controls or an established reference range? How we interpret the results will depend on who the comparison was made with. The difference seen is statistically significant but this may or may not be associated with a clinically important difference – although the fact that the question states that values are 'severely' depleted suggests a clinically relevant reduction has occurred. There may or may not be other factors, such as age, that need to be taken into account when interpreting the results. The study was presumably undertaken to answer some research question, the answer to which would inform clinical practice. Therefore we do not expect to do nothing after obtaining the trial results. On the other hand we do not want to introduce (or even trial) supplementation without first considering the clinical relevance and implications for the reduction found. The *p* value shows that the study is large enough that the observed difference cannot be attributed to chance. Hence, the most correct answer is B.

answers

23. D: Carry out a trial of a larger size to obtain a more precise estimate of the effect of the new diet compared to standard

The average improvement seen is clinically relevant so we would not just want to discount the information because it is statistically non-significant. The confidence interval for the difference is wide and shows that the data are compatible with the new dietary regimen having no effect, or an adverse effect on height, and also with clinically relevant improvements (up to 1.2 sd scores). Because the diet could be associated with a detrimental or zero effect based on the study results, it would not be reasonable to introduce it as standard purely because the average effect is good. The children could be followed for longer to see whether the effect becomes larger and statistically significant but this would not answer the question of whether an improvement can be seen over 2 years. Sd scores are usually normally distributed, so it is unlikely – although not impossible – that non-parametric methods would be needed. The normality of the scores should have been verified prior to parametric testing. A larger trial would enable a more precise estimate of the effect of the new diet over a 2-year period to be obtained and this would be the best course of action (D is the most correct answer).

24. E: Non-parametric analysis of variance comparing medians between groups (Kruskal–Wallis)

The groups are small, so it is likely that parametric methods are not appropriate. Before embarking on a formal analysis of the differences, the haemoglobin measurements should be plotted according to syndrome group. This plot will allow some assessment of the normality of the measurements. Testing between pairs of groups will enable significant differences to be identified but it does rely on multiple tests and the p values obtained will not be valid without adjustment. It would be preferable to perform one overall test of the significance of the differences observed between groups. It may be that the study is not large enough to identify differences of clinical importance and a larger sample is required. This will become apparent from the plot, significance test and confidence intervals.

25. B: They help to ensure that any differences seen are due to the treatment or disease being studied

If there is no control group then it will not be possible to say whether any effects/outcomes seen in the diseased or treated group are due to the disease or treatment. Hence a control group is necessary. If a historical control group (a group previously measured/assessed) is used then we cannot be sure that any difference is not due to factors that have changed over time (for example, improvement in diet or clinical care). Concurrent controls are therefore preferable. Using concurrent controls will remove some of the potential confounders. We want the controls to be similar to the treatment/disease group so that any differences observed are more likely to be causally attributed to the treatment or disease. If the groups are blind to treatment then treatment knowledge does not differ between groups and so this is a similarity that we want to have (where ethically and feasibly possible).

26. D: It allows the CD4 counts of individual children to be compared to what is expected for normal children of that age

A reference range aims to give information on the values of CD4 found among normal non discased children. It consists of a series of centile values. Since CD4 count changes throughout childhood the range should be age-related. In order to construct precise ranges, quite large groups of children will be needed as we are often interested in extreme centiles (the 5th and beyond). Often the 5th centile is used as a cut-off to define abnormality or cause for further investigation. By definition, 5% of normal healthy individuals will lie on or below the 5th centile. Hence the specificity of a test which uses the 5th centile as a cut-off will be 95%; thus, 95% of those without disease (healthy, normal children like those on whom the reference was based) will have values above the 5th centile and will test 'negative'. The sensitivity of a reference range to detect disease will vary according to the disease. The purpose of the reference range is to allow the CD4 counts of individual children to be compared to what is expected for normal children of that age. If the aim was to compare a group of children with disease to a group of non-diseased children then these non-diseased children should be concurrently measured. Reference ranges are not recommended as a substitute for control groups in trials, rather as assessment tools for individual children. The most correct answer is therefore D.

27. B: A regression analysis should be used and the regression coefficient presented with confidence interval

Firstly the data should be plotted in a scatter-plot of IQ against height. The correlation coefficient could be calculated to estimate significance of any observed association. The relationship could be further quantified by regressing IQ scores on height. This will give a measure of the extent to which IQ changes with height and is much more informative than the correlation coefficient alone. The extent to which the two are related is given by the regression coefficient. Presenting the regression coefficient with a confidence interval shows the range of population scenarios the current sample is compatible with. If the confidence interval is wide then we may decide that a larger sample needs to be taken to obtain a more precise estimate of the relationship. The statistical significance of the observed difference is given by the p value. Since the sample are all 7 years old it is unlikely that expressing their heights as sd scores will make any difference to the results. If the children were over a wider age range and we wanted to remove age as a potential confounder in the comparison of IQ and height, then expressing heights as sd scores would do this.

28. SIGNIFICANCE TESTS

1.   B – Paired *t*-test

There are two groups of children (those with pituitary hormone disorders and their age–sex matched control pairs). Hence a two-sample test for comparison between groups is appropriate (two sample *t*-test, paired *t*-test, Mann–Whitney *U*-test, or chi-square). Outcomes are continuous numeric (blood pressure) and it is the within-pair difference that will be analysed (blood pressure for child with disorder, minus blood pressure for age- and sex-matched pair). Hence the test must be appropriate for continuous outcome data (that is, not Chi-square). Since it is within-pair differences that are to be analysed, these are likely to be normally distributed. The appropriate test to use is the paired *t*-test.

2.   H – Chi-square

There are two groups of children (those admitted to intensive care and those who are not). Hence a two-sample test for comparison between groups is appropriate (two sample *t*-test, paired *t*-test, Mann–Whitney *U*-test, or chi-square). Outcome is binary, that is categoric, with two categories (developmentally delayed: yes/no). The proportion with developmental delay is to be compared between those admitted to intensive care or not. The appropriate test for comparing proportions between two groups is chi-square.

3.   D – One-way analysis of variance

There are four groups of children to be compared (from different racial backgrounds). Hence a test for simultaneous comparison between more than two groups is appropriate (one-way analysis of variance, Kruskal–Wallis analysis of variance, or Chi-square). The outcome (blood pressure) is continuous (hence chi-square is not appropriate) and normally distributed and hence parametric testing should be used (eg one-way analysis of variance).

29.   INTERPRETING TRIAL RESULTS

For all sections A cannot be correct. If the new cream is found to be both statistically and clinically significant then this means that the difference observed is unlikely to be due to chance and is also large enough to make it clinically relevant. The study shows the average difference attributable to the new cream must be large enough to be of clinical importance after taking into account all other factors (cost, ease of use, problem associated with introducing new treatment). Hence in this scenario, the new cream should be introduced.

1.   C – A larger study is required to determine whether it is worth introducing the new cream

The difference is statistically significant since the *p* value (< 0.0005) is small. The average fall of 2.4 points on the severity scale is larger than deemed sufficient to be of clinical importance. However, the confidence interval shows that the data are compatible with a difference of between 1.2 and 3.6 points.

An average fall of 1.2 would not be deemed clinically important enough to warrant changing to the new cream. So the data are compatible with outcomes that are synonymous with differing courses of action. For a fall of 1.2 to less than 2 points on average, the cream would not be introduced, whereas an average fall of between 2 and 3.6 would lead to introduction of the cream. A larger study needs to be done to reduce the width of the confidence interval and gain a more precise estimate of the value of the new cream.

2.   **C – A larger study is required to determine whether it is worth introducing the new cream**

The difference is statistically non-significant since the p value (0.23) is not small. The confidence interval shows that the sample data are compatible with an average change of anywhere between a 6 point drop in favour of the new cream and it making the rash 1.2 points worse on average. Hence we cannot discount scenarios that would lead to introduction of the new cream (ie. a fall of between 6 and 2 on average on the severity scale). Neither can we discount the fact that the new cream does not have a clinically important effect (difference may be less than 2 points and the p value and confidence interval both show data are compatible with no difference between creams). Hence a larger study needs to be done to distinguish between differences of clinical relevance and not.

3.   **I – The results cannot be interpreted because the analysis used was inappropriate**

The difference, confidence intervals and p value are the same as in (1). The observed difference is statistically significant but may or may not be of a clinically relevant magnitude. However, the children allocated to the new cream, but not using it, have been combined with those in the other allocation group. Hence the groups are no longer randomly selected. Those that changed treatment from their allocation may differ in some way that biases the results. The data should have been analysed on an intention-to-treat basis (that is, outcomes compared according to allocated group, rather than according to the treatment actually used). This flaw in the analysis makes it impossible to interpret the results as we cannot assess the extent of any bias.

30. DIAGNOSTIC TESTING

The best way to proceed with a question such as this is to construct the 2 × 2 table of screen result against outcome. The data given is as follows:

Nuchal fold abnormal	Miscarriage		Total
	Yes	No	
Yes			100
No			
Total	80		400

1. I – Percentage correctly classified

Equal numbers of those that miscarry have abnormal or normal nuchal fold thicknesses. So, the information given is:

	Miscarriage		Total
Nuchal fold abnormal	Yes	No	
Yes	40		100
No	40		
Total	80		400

And the rest of the table can be completed, thus:

	Miscarriage		Total
Nuchal fold abnormal	Yes	No	
Yes	40	60	100
No	40	260	300
Total	80	320	400

There are 40 who screen positive (abnormal nuchal fold thickness) and subsequently miscarry. A further 260 screen negative and do not miscarry. This gives a total of 300 (40 + 260) out of the 400 (or 75%) who are correctly diagnosed using the test.

Sensitivity is 40/80 = 50%
Specificity is 260/320 = 81%
Positive predictive value is 40/100 = 40%
Negative predictive value is 260/300 = 87%
False positive rate is 60/100 = 60%
False negative rate is 40/300 = 13%
Positive likelihood ratio is 50/(100 − specificity) = 2.63
Negative likelihood ratio is (100 − 50)/specificity = 0.62
Percentage correctly classified is (40 + 260)/400 = 75%
The prevalence of miscarriage is 80/400 = 20%.

2. C – Positive predictive value

Of those who subsequently miscarry, 75 have abnormal nuchal fold thickness. So, the information given is:

Nuchal fold abnormal	Miscarriage		Total
	Yes	No	
Yes	75		100
No	5		
Total	80		400

And the rest of the table can be completed, thus:

Nuchal fold abnormal	Miscarriage		Total
	Yes	No	
Yes	75	25	100
No	5	295	300
Total	80	320	400

Of the 100 women with abnormal nuchal fold values, 75 (or 75%) subsequently miscarry. Hence the positive predictive value is 75%.

Sensitivity is 75/80 = 94%
Specificity is 295/320 = 92%
Positive predictive value is 75/100 = 75%
Negative predictive value is 295/300 = 98%
False positive rate is 25/100 = 25%
False negative rate is 5/300 = 18%
Positive likelihood ratio is sensitivity/(100 – specificity) = 11.75
Negative likelihood ratio = (100 – sensitivity)/specificity = 0.065
Percentage correctly classified is (75 + 295)/400 = 93%
The prevalence of miscarriage is 80/400 = 20%.

answers

3. A – Sensitivity

Of those with abnormal nuchal fold thicknesses, 60 subsequently miscarry. So, the information given is:

	Miscarriage		Total
Nuchal fold abnormal	Yes	No	
Yes	60		100
No			
Total	80		400

And the rest of the table can be completed, thus:

	Miscarriage		Total
Nuchal fold abnormal	Yes	No	
Yes	60	40	100
No	20	280	300
Total	80	320	400

Of the 80 who miscarry, 60 (or 75%) had an abnormal nuchal fold measurement. This is the sensitivity of the test.

Sensitivity is 60/80 = 75%
Specificity is 280/320 = 88%
Positive predictive value is 60/100 = 60%
Negative predictive value is 280/300 = 93%
False positive rate is 40/100 = 40%
False negative rate is 20/300 = 7%
Positive likelihood ratio is 75/(100 − specificity) = 6.25
Negative likelihood ratio is (100 − 75)/specificity = 0.28
Percentage correctly classified is (60 + 280)/400 = 85%
The prevalence of miscarriage is 80/400 = 20%

Index

This index covers Volume I and Volume II. The volumes are indicated by roman numerals, I and II.

index

index

index

index

index

index

index

index

index